# Psychodynamic Approaches to Behavioral Change

# Psychodynamic Approaches to Behavioral Change

Fredric N. Busch, M.D.
Clinical Professor of Psychiatry, Weill Cornell Medical College
Lecturer in Psychiatry, Columbia University Center for
Psychoanalytic Training and Research
New York, New York

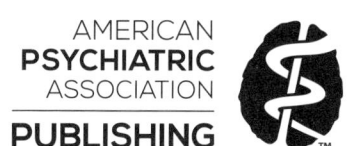

**Note:** The authors have worked to ensure that all information in this book is accurate at the time of publication and consistent with general psychiatric and medical standards, and that information concerning drug dosages, schedules, and routes of administration is accurate at the time of publication and consistent with standards set by the U.S. Food and Drug Administration and the general medical community. As medical research and practice continue to advance, however, therapeutic standards may change. Moreover, specific situations may require a specific therapeutic response not included in this book. For these reasons and because human and mechanical errors sometimes occur, we recommend that readers follow the advice of physicians directly involved in their care or the care of a member of their family.

Books published by American Psychiatric Association Publishing represent the findings, conclusions, and views of the individual authors and do not necessarily represent the policies and opinions of American Psychiatric Association Publishing or the American Psychiatric Association.

If you wish to buy 50 or more copies of the same title, please go to www.appi.org/specialdiscounts for more information.

Copyright © 2019 American Psychiatric Association Publishing
ALL RIGHTS RESERVED
First Edition
Manufactured in the United States of America on acid-free paper
22  21  20  19  18    5  4  3  2  1
American Psychiatric Association Publishing
800 Maine Ave., SW
Suite 900
Washington, DC 20024-2812
www.appi.org

**Library of Congress Cataloging-in-Publication Data**
Names: Busch, Fredric, author.
Title: Psychodynamic approaches to behavioral change / Fredric N. Busch.
Description: First edition. | Washington, D.C. : American Psychiatric Association Publishing, [2019] | Includes bibliographical references and index.
Identifiers: LCCN 2018014207 (print) | LCCN 2018015809 (ebook) | ISBN 9781615372041 (ebook) | ISBN 9781615371303 (pbk. : alk. paper)
Subjects: | MESH: Behavior Therapy—methods | Psychotherapy, Psychodynamic—methods | Problem Behavior—psychology
Classification: LCC RC489.B4 (ebook) | LCC RC489.B4 (print) | NLM WM 425 | DDC 616.89/142—dc23
LC record available at https://lccn.loc.gov/2018014207

**British Library Cataloguing in Publication Data**
A CIP record is available from the British Library.

# Contents

Preface .................................................................. vii

1 Understanding Behavioral Change in Psychoanalytic Treatments ........................................ 1

2 Psychodynamic Understanding of Factors That Impede Behavioral Change .......................... 13

3 Identifying and Addressing Risks in Targeting Behavioral Change ................................................ 27

4 Using Psychodynamic Techniques in Addressing Behavioral Change ............................ 41

5 A Framework for Targeting Behavioral Change .... 55

6 Identifying Dynamic Contributors to Problematic Behaviors ........................................... 73

7 Identifying Alternative Behaviors .......................... 87

8 Identifying Interfering Factors in Performing Alternative Behaviors ........................................... 101

**9** Working With Sustaining Behavioral Change and the Response of Others.................................. 111

**10** Engaging the Patient in Addressing Specific Behavioral Problems............................................. 123

**11** Addressing Behavioral Problems Related to Adverse Developmental Experiences and Trauma................................................................. 141

Index.................................................................. 155

# Preface

Psychoanalysts have avoided emphasizing or targeting behavioral change in psychoanalysis or psychoanalytic psychotherapies, believing such efforts can disrupt or derail effective treatment (Freud 1917/1963, 1923/1955; Gabbard 2014; Greenson 1967). A central concern has been that these strategies constitute "suggestion," an effort to influence or manipulate patients, which Freud (1917/1963) made clear was to be excluded or minimized in psychoanalytic treatments. The predominant focus of psychoanalysts was on gaining insight, making the unconscious conscious; this increased understanding was considered the primary goal, paving the way for behavioral change. If behavioral change occurred without proper analysis, conflicts were believed to persist, leading to the substitution of different symptoms or problematic behaviors. Over the course of psychoanalytic history, there has been an increasing emphasis on the clinical impact of the therapeutic relationship independent of insight, but theories and approaches that expand on this process still consider behavioral change to be a secondary outcome. Although clinical evidence suggests that more psychoanalysts are now targeting behavioral change, published case reports and strategic frameworks have been limited (see Chapter 1, "Understanding Behavioral Change in Psychoanalytic Treatments").

Elucidating unconscious conflicts and a productive therapeutic relationship can contribute to behavioral change, but patients (and people in general) often require additional interventions to modify behaviors. Indeed, behavior frequently proves quite resistant to change, as many factors contribute to the persistence of habitual or reflexive patterns. Other psychotherapeutic schools, such as cognitive-behavioral therapies (Thoma et al. 2015), have developed approaches to target behavioral change, a factor that has contributed to patients pursuing therapies other than psychoanalytic treatments. There are numerous strategies for changing behavior, including (but not limited to) identifying and modifying the context in which the behavior occurs, establishing a basis to consider alternative behaviors, determining signals to remind patients to shift behaviors, engaging different mental states that lead to new behaviors, and systematically desensitizing fears that inhibit behaviors. A component of trial-and-error learning—one that includes ongoing assessment and testing of the impact of changed behaviors—is usually involved.

Rather than being at odds with or disruptive to psychoanalytic treatments, this book demonstrates how efforts to change behavior can be part of the development and employment of a psychodynamic formulation and therapy and can be used to enhance self-understanding and exploration of the transference. Work on behavioral change can improve the therapeutic alliance as therapist and patient collaborate in making practical changes in the patient's life. There are a variety of ways in which efforts at behavioral change can be integrated with and enhanced by psychodynamic exploration. In most instances these approaches can become a core part of the process of understanding and identification of the patient's dynamics, conflicts, and self and object representations.

Psychoanalytic theory and techniques add several strategies for behavioral change to those employed in other treatments. These include exploring unconscious dynamics that are interfering with behavioral change and using the transference to observe conflicts and inhibitions as they emerge with the therapist. Identifying developmental experiences contributing to these conflicts and behaviors aids patients in determining their origins, helping to assess if the risks associated with behaviors have been overestimated based on early experiences. Patients can also come to understand how problematic behaviors may have been previously adaptive. Another crucial component is the capacity to assess countertransference reactions, which can lead therapists to be overly focused on behavioral change, expect that patients follow their advice more readily than they are capable of, or overlook patients' concerns about the value of suggested actions.

From the psychoanalytic perspective, multiple factors are contributory to behavioral problems, and identifying and addressing these various factors aids in change in behavior over time. For example, patients with difficulties with assertiveness may struggle with conflicts regarding their aggression, a fear of disrupting close attachment relationships, and separation fears from increased autonomy. Adverse early experiences, such as harsh punishments of assertive behavior, may have added to the intensity of these fears. The psychodynamic therapist works to address these various contributors in targeting behavioral change. In addition, psychodynamic therapists attend to unsymbolized states (Busch 2017), which include somatic or other internal experiences that are not recognized as being emotional or symbolic. The therapist works with the patient to identify the emotions and fantasies that contribute to these states and to understand their dynamic meaning and impact on behavior.

My interest in psychodynamic approaches to behavioral change arose serendipitously in developing focused psychodynamic approaches to anxiety disorders (Busch et al. 2012) and depression (Busch et al. 2016). In examining why patients receiving these treatments rapidly improved in a short period, I became aware that I was focusing more than usual on behavioral change, often involving difficulties with assertiveness. Understanding the dynamics and conflicts associated with these disorders was very helpful in identifying the contributors to unassertiveness and avoidance. Psychoanalytic understanding could be used to target these behavioral problems, leading to a more rapid resolution of the symptoms and inhibitions. These observations led me to the notion of focusing on behavioral problems as a key element in short-term psychodynamic interventions. I found that the negative view psychoanalysts have had toward targeting behavior has interfered with the development of valuable therapeutic strategies that can increase the rapidity of behavioral change and symptom relief. In fact, psychodynamic approaches are particularly useful in addressing behavioral problems alongside symptoms and characterological difficulties. This book demonstrates to psychodynamic clinicians that they can appropriately target behavioral interventions and provides a framework for clinicians using psychodynamic techniques to enhance behavioral change.

Some background training in psychoanalytic theory and approaches will aid in understanding this book, but it is written to appeal to a broad range of mental health professionals who use a variety of treatment approaches. The material is presented in clear language with limited jargon and many illustrative vignettes. Those with less exposure to psychoanalytic concepts may want to start with Chapter 4, "Using Psychodynamic Techniques in Addressing Behavioral Change," which includes some definitions of basic terms. Otherwise these readers may want to review

Chapter 3, "Basic Psychodynamic Concepts," in *Panic-Focused Psychodynamic Psychotherapy—eXtended Range* (Busch et al. 2012), which defines core psychoanalytic terms and concepts.

Portions of this book, particularly in Chapters 1 and 5, have been adapted, with permission, from an earlier article of mine: "Promoting Behavioral Change in Psychoanalytic Treatments." *Psychodynamic Psychiatry* 45(1):79–102, 2017. Copyright © 2017, Guilford Publications.

## References

Busch FN: A model for integrating actual neurotic or unrepresented states and symbolized aspects of intrapsychic conflict. Psychoanal Q 86(1):75–108, 2017 28272818

Busch FN, Milrod BL, Singer M, et al: Panic-Focused Psychodynamic Psychotherapy—eXtended Range. New York, Routledge, 2012

Busch FN, Rudden MG, Shapiro T: Psychodynamic Treatment of Depression, 2nd Edition. Arlington, VA, American Psychiatric Press, 2016

Freud S: Introductory lectures on psycho-analysis, part III (1917), in The Standard Edition of the Complete Psychological Works of Sigmund Freud, Vol 16. Translated and edited by Strachey J. London, Hogarth Press, 1963, pp 241–463

Freud S: Two encyclopaedia articles (1923), in The Standard Edition of the Complete Psychological Works of Sigmund Freud, Vol 18. Translated and edited by Strachey J. London, Hogarth Press, 1955, pp 233–260

Gabbard G: Psychodynamic Psychiatry in Clinical Practice. Arlington, VA, American Psychiatric Publishing, 2014

Greenson R: The Technique and Practice of Psychoanalysis, Vol 1. Madison, CT, International Universities Press, 1967

Thoma N, Pilecki B, McKay D: Contemporary cognitive behavior therapy: a review of theory, history, and evidence. Psychodyn Psychiatry 43(3):423–461, 2015 26301761

# Understanding Behavioral Change in Psychoanalytic Treatments

This chapter reviews factors that have led psychoanalysts to avoid focusing on behavioral change (Table 1–1) and describes more recent efforts to target behavioral change. Although theorists and clinicians erred in believing that focusing on behavioral change would be inherently damaging to treatment, they identified specific difficulties to be alert to in using these strategies, including potential disruptions in the therapeutic relationship. In recent years, psychoanalysts have described techniques for handling the prescribing of medication, and some clinicians have begun to develop strategies focused on behavioral change. The use of these approaches suggests ways in which targeting behavioral change can aid, rather than disrupt, psychoanalytic goals.

## Why Psychoanalysts Have Avoided Focusing on Behavioral Change

### The Avoidance of "Suggestion"

The historical reaction in psychoanalysis to more directive interventions, such as behavioral change, can be traced to Freud's wish to minimize

**TABLE 1–1. Why psychoanalysts have avoided focusing on behavioral change**

Avoidance of "suggestion": interferes with developing insight
Disruptions of neutrality: suggestions take a side in patients' conflicts
Disruptions in abstinence: behavioral suggestions gratify patients
Symptom substitution: behavioral change requires insight
Disruptions in the therapeutic relationship
    Pressure to be the "good" patient
    Becoming dependent on the therapist
    A need to submit to the therapist
    An urge to rebel against suggestions

the role of suggestion after he revised his early theories and approaches, such as hypnosis. In elaborating on the need to avoid suggestion, Freud (1917/1963) contrasted it with the effort to identify underlying motivations: "Direct suggestion is suggestion aimed against the manifestation of the symptoms; it is a struggle between your authority and the motives for the illness. In this you do not concern yourself with these motives; you merely request the patient to suppress their manifestation in symptoms" (p. 448). Freud (1923/1955) clearly differentiated psychoanalytic approaches as excluding suggestion: "Psycho-analytic procedure differs from all methods making use of suggestion, persuasion, etc., in that it does not seek to suppress by means of authority any mental phenomenon that may occur in the patient" (p. 250).

Despite these concerns, Ferenczi (1921/1980) developed an "active therapy" that sought change through particular behavioral interventions, for example, by encouraging a patient to sing in psychotherapy. Although he noted that these strategies should only be used when the usual psychoanalytic techniques had failed, his ideas were not welcomed by the psychoanalytic community, particularly Freud. As Freud (1924/1965) averred, "active therapy is a dangerous temptation to ambitious beginners" (p. 481). As with many new theories and therapeutic approaches, Freud's antagonism put a damper on further exploration of these strategies. Targeting behavior, including giving advice, eventually was placed under the heading of "supportive" psychotherapy, which was typically seen as inferior to "expressive" or insight-oriented psychodynamic psychotherapy (Gabbard 2014).

## Disruptions in Neutrality and Abstinence

Psychoanalysts have avoided focusing on behavioral change in part because of its perceived disruption of core components of the analyst's stance, neutrality and abstinence, both of which are considered essential to treatment effectiveness. *Neutrality* refers to the analyst's not siding with the ego, superego, or id, aspects of the individual that are often in conflict; the goal is, instead, to help elucidate these various elements. It subsequently has been interpreted to mean that the analyst is neutral with regard to the patient's behavior or choices (Gabbard 2014; Kelly 1998). According to this understanding of neutrality, because a person is in conflict about what action to take, the analyst would not want to take sides by suggesting or advising that the patient behave in a particular way. If the therapist suggests a specific action, then the patient would be in conflict about whether to enact it, or have an urge to do the opposite behavior. Furthermore, encouraging or advising behavioral change may be viewed as gratifying the patient (Gabbard 2014). Gratification, as opposed to the technical stance of abstinence, is believed to interfere with the patient's motivation to explore unconscious intrapsychic conflicts. However, other psychoanalysts have suggested that these technical concepts have been overextended, problematically limiting the analyst's flexibility in treating patients (Busch and Sandberg 2007).

## Symptom Substitution

As noted in the introduction, psychoanalysts generally believe that gaining insight into intrapsychic conflicts is essential to relieve symptoms, inhibitions, and problematic behaviors (Kazdin 1982). If the symptom or behavior was changed without the underlying intrapsychic conflict becoming conscious and being explored, another symptom or problematic inhibition would arise as an expression of the conflict. As cognitive behavioral therapies began to demonstrate that symptoms could be relieved without insight about intrapsychic conflicts (Thoma et al. 2015), clinicians questioned whether this theory was correct. Wachtel (1997) suggested that symptom substitution does not happen in behavioral treatments because patients confront fears in new ways, which may not include gaining insight. Indeed, empirical research thus far suggests that symptom substitution is not a typical occurrence (Tryon 2008).

### Disruptions in the Therapeutic Relationship

Psychoanalysts believe that working directly with behavioral change, with its use of suggestion and distortions in neutrality and abstinence, can lead to the development of problematic patterns in the therapeutic relationship, which can take several forms. Patients, aware that the therapist wants them to make certain changes, could develop a need to please the therapist by trying to change behavior and/or may develop feelings of inadequacy if they are unable to make the change. They may also feel pressured to submit to the therapist's suggestions and view themselves as "bad" patients if they do not follow through or complete the task that they are working on in therapy. Patients could become dependent on the therapist, feeling that they need the therapist's advice to make decisions. Alternatively, as mentioned above, the therapist, by taking a side in a patient's conflicts through giving particular suggestions, could induce a struggle within the patient about whether to follow or rebel against the therapist's suggestions. These distortions can complicate the therapist's interpretation of the transference, a key component of psychoanalytic therapies (see Chapter 4, "Using Psychodynamic Techniques in Addressing Behavioral Change"). In recent years, proponents of targeting behavior have suggested that although it is important to be alert to these risks, positive changes can often enhance the therapeutic relationship.

## The Shifting View on Behavioral Interventions

These concerns about adverse consequences have inhibited psychoanalysts from considering what role they may play in more directly helping patients with behavioral change, leaving them at a loss as to how to proceed theoretically or technically in this effort, other than to avoid it. However, in recent years, psychoanalysts have developed approaches for being prescriptive, such as recommending and treating patients with medications (Busch and Sandberg 2007) or obtaining a treatment contract with agreements about such issues as self-destructive behaviors (Levy et al. 2006). Summers and Barber (2010), describing pragmatic psychodynamic psychotherapy (PPP), addressed the importance of focusing on behavioral change and criticized psychoanalysts for their lack of interest in this area or for presuming that behavioral changes occur "downstream" from insight. They noted how behavioral changes have an impact on emotions and conflicts and may be necessary to produce change in self-perceptions.

### Case Example

Ms. A, a 38-year-old social worker with generalized anxiety disorder and occasional panic attacks, was chronically anxious about tasks she believed she needed to perform for others and was perfectionistic in her efforts to accomplish them. As her responsibilities increased, in part because of the pressure she experienced to say yes to requests for help, her anxiety intensified. For example, she felt it essential to spend considerable time searching for just the right gifts to make others happy for birthdays and holidays, and believed not doing so could be terribly disappointing and hurtful to those others. She was prone to panic attacks when she felt the pressure to make the proper choices or to respond to others when their requests began to increase.

Therapist and patient determined that a major contributor to her anxiety was Ms. A's inability to set a limit on the activities that she consented to. When they explored what she felt when being asked to do certain tasks, such as taking charge of her son's school committee, she became aware of angry feelings but struggled with acknowledging or expressing her anger. The anger included a sense that she was being picked for too many tasks because she was more responsible than others. The conflict about being angry often resulted in the defense of reaction formation (see Chapter 4), in which she would suppress her anger and increase her efforts to take care of others. While exploring these feelings and dynamics, the therapist identified how her perfectionistic responsiveness added to her feelings of intense anxiety. Much of this "people pleasing," as she referred to it, appeared to have started early in life, when she often felt it necessary to take care of her highly anxious parents, rather than be cared for by them. Another contributing factor was feelings of inadequacy, in part related to early fears that she could not actually relieve her parents' distress or get them to appropriately respond to her needs.

Insight into the dynamics and origins of this problematic behavior at first had little impact on it, and there was limited additional progress in exploring her angry feelings, which she continued to minimize. As her panic attacks were clearly related to her inability to control the pressure to respond to others, one goal of therapy, while exploring the dynamics, became helping the patient to reduce these feelings and behavior to a more tolerable level. The therapist made comments suggesting the importance of taking such steps, including the following: "It seems like you need to consider turning down more activities so you don't feel so overwhelmed"; "You work so hard to get the perfect gift that it makes you very unhappy. Maybe you don't have to make such an effort"; and "Maybe if you hold yourself back, we will get more information about why you are so fearful of making the other person upset." The therapist and patient attended to moments when the patient felt compelled to take on a task, including things she might say when asked (e.g., "I would love to take this on, but I have too many other tasks I'm engaged in at this point") and what feelings, fears, and fantasies were triggered at that point.

As Ms. A began to hold back on her usual reflexive tendency to respond, she became more aware of angry feelings she was having about being asked to take on additional tasks for the school when others had taken on far fewer, and toward people who were not doing the jobs they were assigned. She was then able to use this anger to fuel her capacity to say no, overcoming her worries about others and her feelings of insecurity if she did not take on a task. As she began to make these changes, she was relieved to find that others were not damaged or hurt in the way she feared; indeed, sometimes they seemed relieved when she confronted them and accepted their tasks more readily. These steps greatly eased her fears about harming others through limit setting and gave her a feeling of increased effectiveness and empowerment over others, reducing her insecurity and anxiety. The improvement in her self-esteem helped to ease the pressure she felt to please others and get their approval, and reduced the frequency of her panic attacks.

## Psychoanalytic Tools for Addressing Behavioral Change

Despite the focus on insight and proscriptions regarding behavioral interventions, one could argue that psychoanalysts are in a particularly good position to help patients reach decisions or change behaviors in positive or productive ways. Knowledge of the unconscious and of the types of intrapsychic conflicts and personality difficulties that patients struggle with helps therapists to predict and identify the kinds of behavioral problems that might emerge as well as strategies to address them. Analysts can work with patients to elucidate how developmental events, defenses, fantasies, or predominant self and object representations may be interfering with efforts to change specific behaviors. Helping patients in this way is very different from advising them what to do in particular circumstances. The primary aim is to aid patients in identifying behaviors that may help them to better accomplish their goals and factors that can interfere with making productive behavioral choices.

## Analysts' Current Prescriptive Interventions

Although the notion of encouraging behavioral change has been frowned on, psychoanalysts have been increasingly prescriptive in many situations and have developed technical approaches for making these interventions. One area involves recommending, prescribing, and monitoring psychotropic medication (Busch and Sandberg 2007), which studies indicate occurs frequently in psychoanalytic treatment (Doidge et al. 2002; Donovan and Roose 1995). Initially viewed as predominantly damaging to psychoanalysis, the integration of medication treatment and analytic work is now seen as commonplace and primarily helpful (Busch and Sandberg 2007). Adapting theory and technique to manage these interventions (Busch and Sandberg 2007) has included a suggestion that psychoanalysts "switch gears" to a mode in which they assess symptoms and discuss appropriate psychotropic medication and dosing (Cabaniss 1998). They can then return to an analytic mode in attending to dynamics and meanings of symptoms and medications, as well as in exploring how the analyst's efforts in prescribing medication are perceived. In addition to a perspective that considers dynamic factors and one that assesses phenomenology or behavior, therapists should have a "central gear" that allows them to weigh various dynamics (including the state of the transference and countertransference) and phenomenological factors (Busch and Sandberg 2007). Many authors and clinicians (see Busch and Sandberg 2007; Cabaniss 1998; Donovan and Roose 1995) now aver that medication interventions can be accomplished without significantly disrupting analytic treatment.

Such technical approaches are valuable in developing interventions that target behavior. The therapist can consider and address behavioral change and then move to the dynamics related to the behavior and therapeutic relationship. The therapist can relate the dynamics to behavioral interventions, as well as assess transference and countertransference factors that affect the therapist's decision-making process. These strategies will help ensure that the therapist's interventions both encourage behavioral change and advance dynamic exploration.

## Approaches to Behavioral Change in Psychoanalytic Treatments

In signs of a shift to considering targeting behavior directly, psychodynamic clinicians have increasingly discussed both theoretical bases of and clinical approaches to behavior change (Table 1–2). Wachtel (1977) initially focused on this area, exploring the integration of psychoanalysis and behavior therapy, and concluded that there were many areas of overlap between the treatments and an unnecessary antagonism. He believed that behavioral techniques, including assertiveness training or systematic desensitization, could be employed in conjunction with analytic therapy. He emphasized the importance of exploring relationships outside the therapeutic setting and the value of attending to what was occurring in these contexts. It was important to consider, in his view, not only how wishes and conflicts would lead to certain behavioral difficulties, but also how problematic relationships and behaviors can lead to the intensification of certain conflicts.

Wachtel (1977, 2014) described patterns of vicious cycles between intrapsychic states and interactions with others that would maintain psychopathology, such as a depressed individual's expectation of rejection-triggering avoidant or irritable behavior, which can inadvertently lead others to withdraw or become angry. Identifying and interrupting these vicious cycles is important both to relieve internal conflicts and symptoms and improve relationships. For these purposes Wachtel believed it was necessary to more actively intervene in patients' behavioral patterns. To achieve these goals, therapists may need to teach social skills or advise patients on their interpersonal interactions.

Summers and Barber (2010) view behavioral change as an important component of PPP. The initial interventions of this approach are more standard, involving exploration of painful feelings, fantasies, and memories, with further work to develop alternative perspectives on problematic current situations. Therapist and patient then employ these new perspectives to develop alternative responses to these circumstances, in part by using behaviors and social skills derived from areas of their lives less affected by conflict. These behavioral changes have a significant impact on emotions, conflicts, and self-perceptions. The therapist is alert to the risks to the therapeutic relationship discussed above, including being drawn into power struggles, obscuring the transference, infantilizing the patient, or "reproducing earlier traumatic situations by telling a patient what to do" (p. 45), but the benefit of developing new behaviors, in their view, often outweighs these risks. "New behaviors are considered, not pushed" (p. 45), as the therapist monitors the state of the therapeutic alliance. Summers and Barber describe a case in which the therapist and patient developed a set of "scripts" to change a pattern in which the patient took over too many chores for his depressed wife, which enabled him to express concern but not immediately offer help. However, they do not develop an extended framework through which behavioral problems can be systematically targeted.

In time-limited dynamic psychotherapy, or TLDP, developed by Levenson (2010), the therapist and patient identify cyclical maladaptive interpersonal problems and how internal struggles (considered as resulting from these patterns and problematic affects) contribute to these problems, a concept somewhat related to Wachtel's (1977) approach. More typical psychotherapeutic techniques are employed, such as clarification, confrontation, and interpreting the transference, but the therapist focuses on how these problematic interactive patterns have developed from relationships between self and others and what maintains them. The therapist highlights repetitive patterns as they emerge in the transference, in past and present relationships, as well as in self and other representations (e.g., self-criticism). As these problematic interpersonal processes are identified, patients begin to recognize their occurrence in their daily lives. Patients do "homework" in which they practice identifying particular dynamics occurring with others. This new perspective enables them to examine their role in perpetuating dysfunctional interactions and promotes self-observation. Once patients can recognize dysfunctional patterns and link them to emotional states, they can focus on changing them. This growing awareness enables the patient to anticipate opportunities to interact differently.

The formulation of cyclical problematic interpersonal relationships is used to identify new behaviors that will diminish maladaptive patterns and self-views. In addressing efforts at behavioral change, the therapist is aware that patients avoid behavior that triggers shame and anxiety. Experiential learning is emphasized to address these painful feelings, paving the way for new behaviors. Alternative behaviors are, it is hoped, rewarded, allowing for a shift to new patterns and a new experience of self and others. Thus, there is a change in mentalization as the patient becomes more aware of the impact of different behaviors, and a shift to new working models of relationships. The therapist may give directives to help the patient foster his or her growth outside the session, including homework. As with PPP, the therapist using directives is alert to the risk of reenacting a dysfunctional pattern.

Although these authors have made efforts to target behavioral changes, the approaches put forth are either incomplete (Wachtel; Summers and Barber) or highly complex (Levenson). This book will describe a broad framework for targeting behavioral change that addresses these limitations.

## Behavioral Change as an Aid to Psychoanalytic Goals

This book suggests that targeting behavioral change, rather than disrupting the psychoanalytic process, often aids in exploration and in gaining insight (Table 1–2). Examining behavioral difficulties enhances the overall psychodynamic understanding of the patient. Considerable exploration takes place in identifying behaviors that are problematic and factors that inhibit changing these behaviors. Targeting behavioral change provides an opportunity to observe what comes to mind in terms of fantasy, affects, and conflicts when envisioning and enacting these changes, providing additional intrapsychic information that may not have been obtained if these efforts were not made. Working with behavioral change allows for exploration of transferences that emerge in this effort, such as a need to please or defy the therapist, or wishes to be taken care of. Each of these transference reactions can interfere with behavioral change, and exploration of these reactions provides opportunities to work through conflicts about assertiveness, anger, and dependency. Additionally, as will be discussed in Chapter 9 ("Working With Sustaining Behavioral Change and the Response of Others"), changes in behavior allow for confrontation of specific fears and fantasies. For instance, successful assertive behavior can help patients reassess fears that expressing their needs or feelings directly will inherently lead to damage or disruption with others. Thus, these psychoanalytically informed approaches can be valuable for a purpose that has not been a previous focus of exploratory treatments—namely, changing behavior—hence expanding the therapist's armamentarium for helping patients to obtain insight, relieve distress, and improve relationships.

**TABLE 1–2.** Efforts at behavioral change and psychoanalytic goals

Identify problematic behaviors and thereby expand the psychodynamic formulation
Provide information about dynamics
Provide additional information about the transference
Change and diminish intrapsychic conflicts

# References

Busch FN, Sandberg L: Psychotherapy and Medication: The Challenge of Integration. Hillsdale, NJ, Analytic Press, 2007

Cabaniss DL: Shifting gears: the challenge to teach students to think psychodynamically and psychopharmacologically at the same time. Psychoanal Inq 18:639–656, 1998

Doidge N, Simon B, Brauer L, et al: Psychoanalytic patients in the U.S., CANADA, and Australia: I. DSM-III-R disorders, indications, previous treatment, medications, and length of treatment. J Am Psychoanal Assoc 50(2):575–614, 2002 12206544

Donovan SJ, Roose SP: Medication use during psychoanalysis: a survey. J Clin Psychiatry 56(5):177–178, discussion 179, 1995 7737955

Ferenczi S: The further development of the active therapy in psychoanalysis (1921), in Further Contributions to the Theory and Technique of Psycho-Analysis. Edited by Richman J. London, Karnac Books, 1980, pp 198–217

Freud S: Introductory lectures on psycho-analysis, part III (1917), in The Standard Edition of the Complete Psychological Works of Sigmund Freud, Vol 16. Translated and edited by Strachey J. London, Hogarth Press, 1963, pp 241–463

Freud S: Two encyclopaedia articles (1923), in The Standard Edition of the Complete Psychological Works of Sigmund Freud, Vol 18. Translated and edited by Strachey J. London, Hogarth Press, 1955, pp 233–260

Freud S: Letter from Sigmund Freud to Karl Abraham, February 15, 1924 (1924), in The Complete Correspondence of Sigmund Freud and Karl Abraham 1907–1925. Transcribed and edited by Falzeder E. Translated by Schwarzacher C. London, Karnac, 1965, pp 480–483

Gabbard GO: Treatments in psychodynamic psychiatry, in Psychodynamic Psychiatry in Clinical Practice, 5th Edition. Washington, DC, American Psychiatric Publishing, 2014, pp 99–134

Kazdin AE: Symptom substitution, generalization, and response covariation: implications for psychotherapy outcome. Psychol Bull 91(2):349–365, 1982 7071264

Kelly KV: Principles, pragmatics, and parameters in clinical analysis: the dilemma of pharmacotherapy. Psychoanal Inq 18:716–729, 1998

Levenson H: Brief Dynamic Therapy (Theories of Psychotherapy Series). Washington, DC, American Psychological Association, 2010

Levy KN, Clarkin JF, Yeomans FE, et al: The mechanisms of change in the treatment of borderline personality disorder with transference focused psychotherapy. J Clin Psychol 62(4):481–501, 2006 16470612

Summers RF, Barber JP: Psychodynamic Therapy: A Guide to Evidence-Based Practice. New York, Guilford, 2010

Thoma N, Pilecki B, McKay D: Contemporary cognitive behavior therapy: a review of theory, history, and evidence. Psychodyn Psychiatry 43(3):423–461, 2015 26301761

Tryon WW: Whatever happened to symptom substitution? Clin Psychol Rev 28(6):963–968, 2008 18329771

Wachtel PL: Psychoanalysis and Behavioral Therapy: Toward an Integration. New York, Basic Books, 1977

Wachtel PL: Psychoanalysis, Behavioral Therapy, and the Relational World. Washington, DC, American Psychological Association, 1997

Wachtel PL: An integrative relational point of view. Psychotherapy (Chic) 51(3):342–349, 2014 25068191

# 2

# Psychodynamic Understanding of Factors That Impede Behavioral Change

Psychoanalysts have identified many factors that lead to problematic behaviors and interfere with behavioral change. These include developmental and traumatic events, intrapsychic conflicts, defenses, particular self and object representations, personality difficulties, and disruptions in mentalization skills. Addressing these elements with psychoanalytic approaches aids patients in developing the capacity to change behaviors. A common type of behavioral problem, which will be used as an example in this chapter, involves inhibitions in assertiveness, which can be found in many syndromes, including anxious and depressive disorders, as well as Cluster C personality disorders (American Psychiatric Association 2013; Busch et al. 2012, 2016). Although assertiveness can refer to a wide range of behavior, a useful working definition is the capacity to directly and appropriately express one's feelings, beliefs, and opinions to another person.

This chapter will address a variety of psychodynamic factors that inhibit assertiveness (Table 2–1), although this is not intended to be a com-

**TABLE 2–1.** Factors that contribute to behavior problems: unassertiveness as a focus

Developmental factors, including experience of punitive, withholding, guilt-inducing caregivers
Traumatic experiences, including abandonment, loss, abuse
Self and other representations, including viewing the self as weak, inadequate; others as controlling, rejecting
Intrapsychic conflicts, including angry feelings and fantasies triggering fears of damage retaliation
Defense mechanisms, including reaction formation and passive aggression
Personality difficulties, including Cluster C personality disorders
Deficits in mentalization skills

plete list, as a broad array of dynamic constellations can contribute to a behavioral problem. Various elements relevant to a particular patient's mental life, symptoms, and behavioral difficulties are organized in what is referred to as a *psychodynamic formulation* (Perry et al. 1987), which specifies and integrates these factors. The formulation, which is developed over the course of treatment, provides a framework for the use of psychodynamic techniques (see Chapter 4, "Using Psychodynamic Techniques in Addressing Behavioral Change") in targeting symptoms and behavioral change.

# Developmental Factors and Traumatic Experiences

Developmental factors, particularly experiences with caregivers in childhood, commonly play a role in problems with assertiveness; indeed, many patients with disorders associated with unassertiveness report a history of caregivers and others responding in punitive, withholding, or guilt-inducing ways to their attempts to assert themselves (Busch et al. 2012). Individuals internalize such problematic developmental experiences in fantasies or intrapsychic models in which they anticipate others responding in critical or rejecting ways. Traumatic events of abandonment, loss, separation, or abuse can add to a sense of insecure attachment to caregivers, contributing to assertiveness fears, as the individual anticipates that relationships can be easily disrupted or threatened (Allen 2013; Fonagy et al. 1996). These problematic events can lead to the internalization of self and object representations that include a sense of the self as weak, inadequate, and fearful, and a view of others as rejecting or attacking. For instance, a patient with a bullying father was found to have recurrent fantasies in which any effort to assert himself would induce anger in a male authority, who would respond by humiliating and showing him "who was the boss." Some individuals believe assertiveness will harm others, whom they view as weak and easily damaged.

## Intrapsychic Conflicts

Patients with assertiveness problems also tend to struggle with particular intrapsychic conflicts, contradictory and mixed wishes and fantasies, and internalized prohibitions about them (Busch et al. 2012). Such fantasies are typically out of awareness, yet trigger anxiety and guilt; there is an unconscious effort to avert the conscious emergence of a wish or impulse via defense mechanisms (see next subsection). Core conflicts about assertiveness are often linked to angry feelings and impulses, unconsciously linked to assertiveness, with fears of damaging others or causing retaliation or rejection, triggering guilt and anxiety. For instance, the patient referred to earlier experienced rage at authority figures stemming from his father's bullying, which had to be suppressed because his anger was not tolerated. It became evident that the patient confused assertiveness with his own wish to bully and control others, triggering guilt and inhibiting any direct expression of his wishes. Unassertiveness, as with other self-destructive behaviors, may also perform an unconscious self-punitive function in response to underlying guilt, often triggered by intrapsychic conflicts (Markson 1993). A traditional psychoanalytic approach of gaining insight into these dynamics can help to relieve these self-destructive tendencies, but developing alternative assertive behaviors will often aid in this process.

## Defense Mechanisms

Defense mechanisms, characteristic ways in which patients attempt to manage threatening unconscious fantasies or painful affects and perceptions of themselves and others, which can contribute to unassertiveness, include reaction formation and passive aggression (Bloch et al. 1993; Busch et al. 1995, 2012). In *reaction formation* individuals consciously experience and express a feeling opposite to an emotion that is suppressed, such as more positive feelings or behavior toward those with whom they are inwardly angry. With *passive aggression*, frustrations are expressed in an indirect form, such as lateness or withdrawal. These defenses unconsciously attempt to modulate frightening and conflicted feelings and fantasies but interfere with access to and direct expression of frustrations.

## Personality Difficulties

As noted above, unassertiveness is often found in Cluster C personality disorders, including dependent, avoidant, and obsessive-compulsive personality disorders (American Psychiatric Association 2013). Patients with these disorders can demonstrate a heightened sense of dependency, separation fears, shyness, sensitivity to disapproval, avoidance, perfectionism, and overconscientiousness. They often have difficulty tolerating angry feelings and fantasies and struggle with fears of separation and autonomy, interfering with assertiveness. These personality factors should be addressed alongside the other psychodynamic factors contributing to behavioral problems.

## Mentalization Deficits

Patients with unassertiveness often struggle with deficits in *mentalization*, the capacity to conceive of and interpret behaviors and motives in self and others in terms of mental states (Busch 2008; Fonagy and Target 1997). A measure that has been developed to assess this capacity is *reflective functioning* (RF) (Fonagy 2008), which has been found to be significantly associated with various aspects of mental health. For instance, a high level of RF in parents is associated with better mental health in their children (Steele and Steele 2008), and individuals with higher levels of RF who have experienced abuse are less likely to develop borderline personality disorder (Fonagy et al. 1996). Mentalization is most likely to be disrupted in the context of intense attachment relationships, which can impair the ability to communicate needs and wishes. In addition to the capacity to observe the self, understanding the minds, feelings, and motives of others is relevant to behavioral change. Many problematic behaviors occur in response to a misinterpretation of the behavior of others, or anticipation of certain behaviors. An improved comprehension of the motives and communication of others can aid in behavioral change. For instance, Ms. B, whose case is discussed below, feared retaliation from her mother when the patient wanted to express her wishes, but felt less threatened when she recognized that her mother was also struggling with feelings of being pressured by others.

The following vignette describes the identification of contributors to unassertiveness and synthesis of a psychodynamic formulation, aiding in developing approaches to ameliorating these factors and targeting more assertive behaviors.

## Case Example

Ms. B, a 25-year-old graduate student, struggled with assertiveness in a variety of contexts and feared if she pushed for what she wanted it would greatly upset others. In the context of planning her wedding, she experienced trouble asserting her own needs and wishes about various aspects of the ceremony. In particular, her maternal aunt and mother pressed her about certain things they wanted, and she felt pressure to yield, consistent with her other struggles. An initial point of contention was where to have the ceremony, and she accepted their wish to have it in a church, although she preferred a nonreligious venue. Her aunt was covering much of the cost, adding to her guilt about her own wishes and urge to accede to their demands.

In exploring these pressures, it emerged that her concerns were connected developmentally and emotionally to her parents' focus on appearances and achievement, often to the exclusion of empathy with their children. Her mother pushed her to be thin, although the patient was not overweight, and her father compelled her and her brother to perform extremely well academically. Her parents felt it was important to present to the community an appearance that everything was going well with the family, and this focus persisted despite the onset of considerable financial problems that affected their lifestyle. These problems led to a move from a relatively large home to a small apartment at age 14, where she and her younger brother temporarily had to share a room. When the patient complained to her parents about these circumstances, they became angry and responded that she was being selfish, as they often reacted when she expressed frustrations. She developed a pattern of minimizing her own concerns, yielding to both the family's silence with others, their angry reactions toward her, and her own embarrassment about these difficulties. She felt guilty and blamed herself for "making a big deal about her circumstances when others had it far worse." Her parents increasingly fought and got divorced when she was 16.

Developing a psychodynamic formulation, the therapist and patient identified multiple factors contributing to her unassertiveness, including significant developmental stressors surrounding pressures about her appearance and academic performance, a history of being criticized for "complaining," and a shameful need to keep secrets about the family's problems. In this context, she developed a view of herself as "bad" and a "complainer" if she pursued her own wishes. Her intrapsychic conflicts surrounded fantasies about expressing her hurt and angry feelings, which triggered guilt and anxiety about potentially causing a negative impact on others. Her rage at her parents, considered unacceptable, became directed inward and was expressed in self-punitive and self-demeaning ways. This dynamic, common to depression,[1] also interfered with assertiveness and expression of needs as it added to her feelings of inadequacy: she did not believe she deserved attention from others.

Typical defenses included denial of wishes, needs, and angry feelings, as well as reaction formation, in which she took care of others with whom she was inwardly angry. In addition, her mentalization skills were disrupted, as she did not feel able to consider what might be motivating others' controlling behavior. Goals of therapy included helping the patient decide and express what she wanted without experiencing intense guilt and fear of harming others. The therapist addressed these factors and used the formulation to discuss other ways she might respond to her mother and aunt.

> Ms. B: My mother and aunt aren't mean about it, but they were saying we should have a jazz band. I don't want this kind of band and my friends certainly aren't going to like it. I said no, but they just kind of kept pushing it.
> Therapist: Well, given that it's your wedding, why do you feel you need to have the band they want?
> Ms. B: I guess because my aunt's paying for it, and I don't want to disappoint her and my mother. They're being so insistent.
> Th: I think it's important for us to consider your taking a stance on this. It feels as if yielding to this is typical for the pattern in which you feel you must give up your needs to others. However, you end up feeling that you've lost part of yourself and get frustrated and depressed.
> Ms. B: I noticed that I've gotten kind of withdrawn. It's starting to feel like it's not really my wedding. I would really like to stand up to this barrage, but I'm not sure I can do it.

---

[1] See Busch et al. 2016.

> Th: As part of your reaction to these situations, you typically feel powerless and guilty. This is reminiscent of when your family ran into financial problems and told you not to tell anyone. You felt alone, ashamed, and helpless, and I think underneath deeply resentful, but that's not how things need to be now.
>
> Ms. B: It does feel very much like how I felt then. I think we'll really have to work on this. I feel relieved in one way hearing this idea, but then I also feel guilty and frightened.
>
> Th: What frightens you?
>
> Ms. B: I know my mother's going to get upset if I put up resistance to this plan. She'll get very nervous about how her sister will react.
>
> Th: It seems like you are really fearful about hurting her.
>
> Ms. B: I guess so.

The psychodynamic formulation aided both the therapist and the patient in identifying her struggle with setting limits with her aunt and mother. In addition, suggesting a potential behavior to the patient furthered the development of the formulation and the understanding of the patient: The patient's concern about her mother's fragility had not emerged previously.

The fantasies and intrapsychic conflicts involving fear and guilt about damaging others if she expressed her concerns or wishes similarly emerged with her fiancé, Jim, as the therapist targeted addressing her frustrations with him:

> Ms. B: I've been irritated with Jim not supporting me more in these disagreements with my mother. In fact, his parents are also creating pressure about some parts of the wedding, and they're bothering me about it. But I don't want to upset him by bringing them up because he's so excited: He expects it to be so magical.
>
> Th: What problem do you think it will create for him if you ask for more support?
>
> Ms. B: If all I do is complain I think it will ruin it for him.
>
> Th: Well I'm not sure you're at risk of complaining all the time. This sounds like your tendency to be self-critical when you get in touch with your own wishes. How you were always viewed as a "complainer."
>
> Ms. B: I guess the truth is that I'm really disappointed that he won't at least deal with his family, especially with my feeling so stressed by my mother and aunt.

Th: I think the conflict about discussing things with him is the same fear we talked about when dealing with your mother and your aunt. You feel your own needs and anger aren't okay or are harmful to others and that it's not okay to express them.

Ms. B: Well I really do think I'll ruin his happiness about it.

Th: That's part of what I'm saying. That rather than think about how you might discuss your feelings with him and how he might respond, you're focused on how it would hurt him. It's like things felt with your mother and aunt, that it would upset them if you pushed what you wanted for your wedding. It's also the way you felt with your parents growing up. In fact, when you've discussed issues with Jim in the past, he's been quite responsive. The idea that you would ruin his happiness seems like catastrophic thinking.

Ms. B: I guess that's true. It's part of why I'm glad I'm marrying him. We should probably discuss this problem more, and he should talk with his parents. But maybe it's my fault. I should have set better limits from the start about what I wanted for the wedding.

Th: But here again you end up blaming yourself, this time for others' being intrusive or demanding. Your anger gets turned toward yourself.

Ms. B: That's true. It's not my fault his parents started to make demands. I do feel better about this though, and I want to talk to him.

As noted above, Ms. B also struggled with a disruption in mentalization capacities. For example, she would focus on identifying what she did wrong that caused her mother to attack her and did not feel safe reflecting on her mother's mind. However, she was capable of thinking about the minds of others when the relationship and circumstances were less fraught. As described in the dialogue that follows, examining what was going on emotionally and psychologically with her mother was highly valuable for addressing her assertiveness struggles. Ms. B was troubled by pressures from her mother to get together frequently with her stepfather and his children.

Ms. B: I still don't understand why we need to get together with my stepfamily. We're not that close. I don't mind my stepfather, but I find him pushy and controlling. I don't really enjoy their company. Yet my mother keeps insisting that we get together. I saw them at Thanksgiving. Now she wants to spend the day on Christmas!

Th: Have you talked to her about it?

Ms. B: I've tried to say some things, but I think it's just going to make trouble. Also I think she may feel pressured by him.

Th: Tell me about that.

Ms. B: Well he seems kind of insistent. And she says, "What am I supposed to do? I don't want to hurt him and his family." And then I start to get down on myself, thinking "What's the big deal if we see them?"

Th: There are a couple of problems with just accepting this get together without addressing it. You don't really like to visit them during holidays, and keeping that to yourself just maintains your frustration and unhappiness. And you don't really feel you have much of a say in the matter. Your own wishes aren't being taken into account. And we know that's upsetting for you. In other families a mother might say, "Look I understand that melding families is a difficult thing. How do you feel about seeing them again? What compromises can we come up with about activities?" But she doesn't do that.

Ms. B: Yes I know that, but I end up feeling like I'm hurting my mother and being like a bratty child.

Th: We have to say that this is part of an old story. You end up feeling like the bad one. You've always felt that your needs created a problem, and you were "bad" for having them and expressing them. Therefore you end up keeping them to yourself. However, you ultimately get depressed and frustrated because you accept things that you don't want.

Ms. B: Yes, but there's nothing bad about him. He cares about my mother. But he does seem to want to be in control. He wants to be the one to make the decisions.

Th: Well I think that's a problem. And no, he's not bad in the sense that he's not mean to you. But the fact that he's not concerned about your wishes in regard to these visits is a problem.

Ms. B: So then my mother wanted to invite them to my birthday party! I got mad but I didn't want to have a fight. So I nicely said no, but I feel guilty about it, and she seems worried.

Th: I think this shows another aspect of the dynamic that occurs with them and has always happened with your parents. You feel guilty not only because you feel your needs are bad or create trouble for others, but also I think you feel guilty about being angry. Somehow it's not okay. You end up expressing anger toward yourself, being self-critical.

Ms. B: It's true that I felt guilty right after I got mad. But I know before when I've expressed anger my mother gets very upset and we really don't get anywhere. But now I recognize that she's under pressure herself. I said, "You seem really worried about what he thinks." She didn't say much, but it seemed better than prior discussions we've had.

Th: I think it's very useful that you've identified what's going on inside your mother's mind. Maybe it's not so much that you're "bad" but that she's struggling with her own feelings. She feels threatened.

Ms. B: That's a good point. I hadn't really thought about it in that way.

Her increasing awareness of her mother's internal pressure to respond to her stepfather, using her mentalizing capacity, helped her to gain perspective on why her mother attacked her, and contrasted with the belief that the patient was behaving in a hurtful manner. From this perspective, the problems with her assertiveness came in part from the pressure her mother felt, rather than the patient's wish to set limits or get her own needs met. This information also aided in reducing her anger and increasing empathy for her mother, as Ms. B could understand that her mother was dealing with her own sensitivity and anxiety, in which Ms. B became involved secondarily. This better understanding of her own anger and her mother's difficulties helped to ease the patient's guilt.

This increased use of mentalization allows consideration of other ways of approaching the mother about problems. Typically, when Ms. B would finally assert herself, she would express more direct frustration, such as "I don't understand why we have to get together so often," and her mother would get mad at her. Using the information about her mother's reactions, the therapist suggested she might say the following: "It's terrible you feel so much pressure for everything to go just right with him and his family. You're so worried about it. Do you think that's causing you to push me to get together with them?" The mother may be able to have a discussion at this point about her worries. In this case Ms. B may be able to ease her mother's anxiety, thereby relieving pressure on herself. Or her mother may be unwilling to engage in such a discussion, in which case Ms. B would need to set limits on exposure of herself to the mother's adverse impact.

In some cases, a patient may want to suggest to the other person that she consider seeking therapy to relieve stress. The therapist and Ms. B decided to propose that Ms. B stop by briefly on the holiday, which she and her mother agreed to.

> After Ms. B had success in setting up a brief get together, it went relatively well. However, this positive development triggered further guilt, and additional opportunity to work on her conflicts and inhibitions.
>
> Ms. B: So it didn't go as badly as I thought. Then I felt guilty for complaining so much.
> Th: What do you mean by complaining?
> Ms. B: Having expressed so much frustration about getting together. And for saying I don't like my stepfather.
> Th: To your mother?
> Ms. B: No. To Jim. But I still feel it wasn't okay. Later my mother wanted to know how it went, and it was like I was supposed to say how great it was. I just said it was fine.
> Th: You know it's interesting because I know you're capable of expressing frustration with others and joking about situations in other settings. So sometimes expressing your needs is okay. But when it comes to your mother it's very difficult. You've often felt guilty about raising your concerns, even in this instance where your mother accepted them.
> Ms. B: Yes that's true. But I still think she wasn't happy about it.

Here, the therapist refers to a relevant dynamic in which behavioral problems vary according to the context and may be most prominent with close attachment relationships. The intense feelings involved in these relationships increase intrapsychic conflicts and disrupt mentalization skills. The therapist can help patients identify their capacities in less fraught circumstances and then describe how they become disrupted or are not accessible in situations with certain friends or family members. Patients can use this information as part of a framework to reconsider problematic behaviors with close attachment figures. In addition, within a given attachment relationship therapists can identify circumstances that trigger increased conflicts and behavioral difficulties. For Ms. B this contrast could also be made with her fiancé, with whom she had more capacity to express disagreements and felt a limitation in fewer contexts, as in the example noted above.

In exploring the origins of problematic behavior, psychodynamic psychotherapy can identify many contributors to the persistence of these difficulties, including developmental factors, traumatic events, intrapsychic conflicts, defenses, and self and object representations. A psychodynamic formulation that identifies these factors provides a framework to determine and implement alternative behaviors, using the techniques described in subsequent chapters. Behavioral changes will shift patterns with regard to the patient's conflicts and defenses. Thus, rather than being at odds, targeting behavioral changes and identifying contributory psychodynamic factors work conjointly in addressing patients' behavioral problems and symptoms.

# References

Allen JG: Restoring Mentalizing in Attachment Relationships. Arlington, VA, American Psychiatric Publishing, 2013

American Psychiatric Association: Diagnostic and Statistical Manual of Mental Disorders, 5th Edition. Arlington, VA, American Psychiatric Association, 2013

Bloch AL, Shear MK, Markowitz JC, et al: An empirical study of defense mechanisms in dysthymia. Am J Psychiatry 150(8):1194–1198, 1993 8328563

Busch FN (ed): Mentalization: Theoretical Considerations, Research Findings, and Clinical Implications. Hillsdale, NJ, Analytic Press, 2008

Busch FN, Shear MK, Cooper AM, et al: An empirical study of defense mechanisms in panic disorder. J Nerv Ment Dis 183(5):299–303, 1995 7745383

Busch FN, Milrod BL, Singer M, et al: Panic-Focused Psychodynamic Psychotherapy—eXtended Range. New York, Routledge, 2012

Busch FN, Rudden MG, Shapiro T: Psychodynamic Treatment of Depression, 2nd Edition. Arlington, VA, American Psychiatric Press, 2016

Fonagy P: The mentalization-focused approach to social development, in Mentalization: Theoretical Considerations, Research Findings, and Clinical Implications. Edited by Busch F. Hillsdale, NJ, Analytic Press, 2008, pp 3–56

Fonagy P, Target M: Attachment and reflective function: their role in self-organization. Dev Psychopathol 9(4):679–700, 1997 9449001

Fonagy P, Leigh T, Steele M, et al: The relation of attachment status, psychiatric classification, and response to psychotherapy. J Consult Clin Psychol 64(1):22–31, 1996 8907081

Markson ER: Depression and moral masochism. Int J Psychoanal 74(Pt 5):931–940, 1993 8307700

Perry S, Cooper AM, Michels R: The psychodynamic formulation: its purpose, structure, and clinical application. Am J Psychiatry 144(5):543–550, 1987 3578562

Steele H, Steele M: On the origins of reflective functioning, in Mentalization: Theoretical Considerations, Research Findings, and Clinical Implications. Edited by Busch F. Hillsdale, NJ, Analytic Press, 2008, pp 133–158

# Identifying and Addressing Risks in Targeting Behavioral Change

Although this book emphasizes the value of targeting behavioral change in the context of psychodynamic psychotherapy, psychoanalysts have identified certain problems in these approaches that the clinician should be on the alert for. Psychoanalysts have eschewed such approaches rather than recognize that proper monitoring of these factors can help to avert problems arising from them. These difficulties should be considered in any therapy that addresses behavioral change. They include potential adverse impact on the therapeutic relationship, complexities in suggesting particular behaviors, and countertransference factors (Table 3–1). This chapter describes approaches that will limit their possible repercussions, including anticipating and addressing transference reactions and establishing a collaborative stance (Table 3–2).

**TABLE 3–1.** Potential problems in targeting behavioral change

Adverse impact on the therapeutic relationship
    Dependency on the therapist and need to please him or her
    Struggle with the therapist
    Rebellious response to the therapist
Having only the patient's perspective
Countertransference factors
    The therapist's own intrapsychic conflicts
    Frustration with patients' difficulties making changes
    The therapist taking on a paternalistic role

# Adverse Impact on the Therapeutic Relationship

## Dependency on the Therapist

As noted in Chapter 1 ("Understanding Behavioral Change in Psychoanalytic Treatments"), psychoanalysts have identified that working with behavioral change can trigger certain problematic patterns in the therapeutic relationship. Patients, aware that the therapist is encouraging them to modify their actions, can develop a need to please the therapist by trying to make changes, along with feelings of inadequacy if they are unable to. Patients can become dependent on the treatment, as they can develop the view that they need the therapist to advise them on what to do in their lives. Therapists may take on a parental or paternalistic role in patients' lives, potentially adding to patients' difficulties in making their own decisions. In addition, patients may feel pressured to submit to the therapist's suggestions, and view themselves as "bad patients" if they do not follow through or complete the task that they are working on in therapy. Patients can react defiantly or passive aggressively if they do not want to follow the suggestion or if the potential behavior makes them uncomfortable or frightened. Behavioral recommendations can also trigger rebellious urges in patients who are prone to them for various reasons, including difficulties with authority.

In practice, behavioral interventions do not necessarily lead to these problematic relationship patterns. For example, in studies of cognitive-behavioral treatments patients typically become more capable and less

**TABLE 3–2.** Approaches to risks in targeting behavioral change

Working with the transference
Being aware of having only the patient's perspective
Remaining alert to countertransference reactions
Establishing a collaborative approach

symptomatic, rather than more dependent on the therapist (Thoma et al. 2015). However, these studies rarely monitor whether patients struggle with meeting treatment expectations or feel pressured to please the therapist.

To the extent that the therapeutic relationship is affected by targeting behavioral change, psychodynamic psychotherapy provides approaches for addressing these problems. The therapist can point out that the patient will have a variety of reactions to behavioral suggestions, including feelings and wishes toward the therapist, some of which may be troublesome. Exploring these feelings in the context of the transference can aid in resolving these potential problematic reactions. The therapist will be on the alert for reactions such as the patient hoping the therapist will make decisions for them, wishing to please the therapist, or having urges to rebel against suggestions. The therapist should acknowledge that she does not have definitive knowledge of what actions the patient should take in his life and that changing behaviors is a complex task. Such an approach can help reduce the risk of the patient feeling pressured or compelled by the therapist to make changes.

In the following case example, a patient's requests for specific advice were derived in part from conflicted dependent and angry feelings toward authorities (Busch and Milrod 2015). Although the therapist made specific behavioral suggestions, he also addressed how the patient's view of himself as incapable played a defensive role.

### Case Example

Mr. C, a 23-year-old computer technician who reported symptoms of panic attacks, separation anxiety, and depression had failed to respond to several trials of antidepressant medications and psychotherapies. He struggled to move forward in his life, referring at times to being enveloped in a "fog," in which he felt confused and disconnected. He reported being angry about constantly being berated by his female boss and his girlfriend and about being expected to respond immediately to his girlfriend's requests for help. However, he felt unable to counter these attacks and demands, fearing that expressing his anger would cause a loss of these relationships, which exacerbated his separation fears. He also viewed these women as fragile and worried that his angry feelings might hurt them. These relationships paralleled that with his mother, whom he described as punitive and critical to the point of being abusive. He similarly struggled with fears that his anger would lead his mother to be rejecting, or that his rage might damage her. His father was disengaged from the patient and the family conflicts, providing little support. Notably, in his prior treatments, he had avoided telling therapists that he was not feeling helped, not wanting to upset them.

On exploration, Mr. C described that his irritation toward his boss and girlfriend would steadily build when he felt criticized and then shift suddenly to feelings of sadness and inadequacy, or to the state of "fog." Thus, he appeared to unconsciously shut down his rage to prevent expressing it. He believed that if he avoided getting angry, the women would be nice to him. The therapist pointed out that this approach seemed to be a fantasy and was not working. After exploring his anger more directly in this session, Mr. C missed the next two sessions and was very late for the third, becoming confused about the time of the appointment. The therapist interpreted that addressing his rageful feelings had triggered a "fog" regarding therapy. Sharing a preliminary psychodynamic formulation, the therapist suggested Mr. C felt guilty about his anger and directed it toward himself, seeing himself as bad or inadequate. He experienced his emotional needs as unacceptable, leading him to yield to the needs of others, and his acceptance of their criticism was in part a punishment for his wishes and anger. When his irritation and fears became stronger, the "fog" was triggered in a defensive manner. In the following dialogue the therapist initially withheld specific behavioral suggestions, as he was trying to determine if the patient did not know how to assert himself or was just fearful of doing so, and needed to present himself as incompetent.

> Therapist: I think we need to understand why you see yourself as helpless and incapable of addressing your frustrations with others.
> Mr. C: I'm hoping you can give me some specific instructions about what I might say to them.
> Th: I think as we understand more about these feelings you'll get a better idea.
> Mr. C: I really have no idea how to do this. I never had any role models for asserting myself. I don't understand why you can't give me more specific advice.

> Th: I think you're experiencing me as being neglectful like your parents, and may be more capable than you believe.
>
> Mr. C: That is like telling your child who needs help with math to go work on his homework.
>
> Th: Well I think it's good you're able to express this annoyance directly toward me.

This exchange showed an increasing comfort level in revealing frustration toward the therapist, using the transference as a safe opportunity to test his expression of these feelings. As Mr. C began to understand that his anger might not be as damaging as he thought, he made increased efforts to communicate his irritation more directly. He surprised himself and the therapist when he told his boss that she could criticize his work, but it was not okay to insult him. Rather than the feared disruption, his boss behaved less judgmentally toward him. The therapist noted how Mr. C was able to capably confront his boss, which was inconsistent with his self-view of helplessness and incompetence. The therapist raised the possibility that he might similarly assert himself with his girlfriend:

> Th: Now that you were able to set limits with your boss, I'm wondering if you might do the same with your girlfriend.
>
> Mr. C: How do I do that?
>
> Th: It's interesting you ask that, because with your boss you were more capable than you thought.
>
> Mr. C: Well, with my girlfriend it's much scarier.
>
> Th: What do you see as scarier about confronting her?
>
> Mr. C: Oh, I think she's much more likely to be furious or leave. I can't even think of anything I might say.

After several additional sessions the patient still struggled with identifying ways to directly address problems with his girlfriend. Exploration revealed that now that he had confronted his boss he feared he might cross a line, triggering the rejection and retaliation he feared. Additionally, the intimate relationship he shared with his girlfriend had a stronger emotional link to his mother, whose fragility and irritability frightened him. The therapist determined it would be useful at this point to make specific suggestions.

> Mr. C: I understand what you're saying about why I'm so frightened about confronting my girlfriend. But when I'm with her I'm still stuck. Maybe we can talk more about how I might approach her.
>
> Th: Well, what if you said: "I can't always drop everything when you need me, it's just not fair to me or my friends."

> Mr. C: Should I say that? It does sound like a good way of saying that. I don't know how she'll react.
> Th: Well, I think we can talk about it more and try to understand why it's so threatening, especially because you're so upset about these demands.
> Mr. C: Well, I immediately think if I say that she'll get furious and storm out. Very scary. But now that I think about it I'm not sure she would do that. And if she did, I think she would come back.

The therapist's specific suggestion allowed them to explore dangers, including abandonment fears, that emerged if he made the proposed statement to her, a technique described further in Chapter 8 ("Identifying Interfering Factors in Performing Alternative Behaviors"). Following the exploration of this suggestion and others, the patient began more directly to address problems with his girlfriend.

In this context the therapist remained alert to the patient's dependent wishes. In part, the patient's presentation of incompetence was a defensive maneuver to avoid asserting himself, which he viewed as dangerous. At the same time he also struggled with how to appropriately address problems in his most intimate relationships. Interpreting these dynamics along with identifying specific behavioral interventions helped to limit his dependency and increase his assertive behavior.

## Patients in Conflict About the Therapist's Suggestions

The notion that patients will do the opposite behavior from what the therapist suggests, or feel a need to submit to the therapist's recommendation, is a possible but not necessary outcome of a behavioral intervention. Discussing behavioral change can trigger intrapsychic conflicts and certain transference reactions, leading the patient to be unconsciously or consciously resistant or yielding to a therapist's suggestions. In the context of a positive therapeutic alliance, however, the patient typically seeks the therapist's assistance and is not opposed or submissive to potential strategies. The therapist can assess how the patient is responding to these interventions, monitoring for resistance. The sudden development of an unwillingness on the patient's part to consider the suggestion of the therapist or a rapid acceptance could be identified and communicated to the patient and employed as a basis for further exploration. For instance, when treating panic with agoraphobic symptoms, the therapist should explore a patient's unwillingness to expose themselves to feared situations, despite its being a goal of the treatment (Busch et al. 2012).

A patient may also resist a suggestion because he or she believes it may be detrimental, but may be uncomfortable telling the therapist. The therapist should make clear that feedback in response to any recommendation is useful, as the therapist's assessment may indeed be incorrect or may be uncomfortable for the patient to consider. In addition, feedback presents an opportunity to explore the patient's transferential reactions to these interventions, including antagonistic or submissive aspects. In this way behavioral interventions can create opportunities for exploration of the transference.

### Case Example

Mr. D, a 36-year-old financial analyst, chronically struggled with asserting himself at his job, feeling bullied by a younger colleague whom he feared was trying to take over his position. The colleague would criticize him and say negative things about him to their boss. However, he feared directly confronting her because he thought his anger might cause her extreme distress or lead to a problematic altercation, and he worried that he would end up losing his job like his father did; his father had escalated an issue with a colleague at his office and lost the battle. At the same time he believed that he had to be "tough" and manly like his father, but felt weak and damaged by his father's temper growing up. He fantasized about screaming at the colleague that she was incompetent, but then felt inadequate because he held back from making any comment to her. The therapist suggested that the patient viewed these situations as all or none: either he intended to aggressively confront her or would say nothing at all. There seemed to be many alternatives to consider in between.

At that point, Mr. D became angry at him, saying that the therapist was trying to weaken him from taking a firm stance. This led to an opportunity to explore and interpret negative transferences to the therapist: that the therapist might try to competitively undermine him, or was weak and would thereby weaken him. This experience helped illuminate his view of his father as on the one hand manly, impulsive, and temperamental, but also as fearful and insecure. Expressing his pent-up anger at the therapist was a breakthrough for the patient, helping him to feel safer with its expression in general. He then became interested in discussing new ideas about what to say to the colleague, leading to a fruitful discussion about what approach might be best.

## Rebellious Response to Therapist

Sometimes patients may quickly rebel against behavioral suggestions made by the therapist because of intrapsychic conflicts or personality issues. Additionally, patients may respond adversely to a suggestion because it triggers a significant degree of discomfort, guilt, or anxiety. As with other reactions, the therapist can note that the intent is not to pressure the patient to perform the behavior but rather to explore the origins of the patient's response.

### Case Example

Mr. E, a 42-year-old accountant, presented with the onset of depression, as he struggled with pressures to increase the number of clients in his practice; his financial intake was inadequate for him and his family's needs. His symptoms of depression responded fairly well to an antidepressant, but he continued in therapy to address his anxiety and conflicts about his efforts to expand his practice. Although he was deeply worried about his financial circumstances, he tended to get infuriated when others made suggestions for finding new clients, although he feared expressing these feelings. He felt the urge to criticize them, sometimes directly, but usually in an angry preoccupation that the suggestion was "stupid" or "way off the mark." At other points he avoided pursuing certain suggestions or unconsciously "forgot" to follow up on them. Contributors to this defiant tendency included a sense of unfairness and anger about "insiders" and "outsiders," believing that he was an "outsider" who was going to be unfairly rejected by new clients no matter what the circumstances. He felt that others who had connections would automatically get new clients, even when he demonstrated superior skills.

Additionally, he believed that he was unable to work harder because he was prone to anxiety and depression, especially when he had a large number of clients, and that others' expectations were unfair. He stated that he was miserable when he was working long hours and that others should recognize the impact of undue stress on him. His anger often focused on his wife, whom he viewed as hounding or threatening him to increase his clientele, with little empathy about the anxiety and frustration he experienced under these circumstances. As with others, he could not safely express his angry feelings toward his wife, anticipating that he would be attacked or rejected. Thus his rebellion often took place in a defensive, passive aggressive form.

To the extent that the therapist explored how Mr. E could search for additional clients, addressing the fears, frustrations, and feelings of unfairness that interfered with his pursuit, Mr. E felt the urge to rebel, tending to view the therapist as pressing him to work and not recognizing his anxieties and frustrations. Mr. E questioned him in this regard:

> Mr. E: So are you not concerned about whether I can handle having more clients?
> Th: Yes I'm concerned, but I know we're treating your depression and I'm hopeful you will be able to work more. We will also address the concerns you have about it.
> Mr. E: Well, I'm not sure if anyone's adequately recognizing my worries. Everyone just wants me to make money.
> Th: Does that include me?
> Mr. E: Well, yes to some extent. I have to pay for the treatment.
> Th: Well, I think we want to get a sense of why you think I would take a stance that you would feel is unempathic and put my own interest ahead of yours. It seems to trigger rebellious feelings and a wish to hold back on increasing your business. Overall I think you feel better about yourself when you are working more, not to mention that the money is an important issue.
> Mr. E: Okay, well that makes sense. I feel like a loser when I'm not making enough money.

Here the therapist uses the transference—the patient's sense that the therapist's self-interest will override his empathy for Mr. E—to explore his fears of being pushed to make money rather than to be helped. The patient was able to compare the therapist's behavior to what he anticipated from others, including his father's high expectations when he was growing up. This paved the way to identify his angry rebellious urges toward what he assumed was a lack of care for his well-being.

## Other Pitfalls to Be Alert to in Encouraging Behavioral Change

Under any circumstances, a therapist encouraging particular behaviors is a complex matter. Psychotherapists in general may shy away from advising potential behaviors because a problematic outcome may lead patients to be angry and undermine the therapy. A hypothetical example would be a therapist encouraging a patient to confront his boss about mistreatment, only to have the patient return and report that he had been fired. A therapist advising a patient to marry a particular person could later be haunted by this recommendation in the context of significant marital problems or a divorce.

One major problem that can lead to errors in suggesting particular behaviors is that the therapist typically only has information from the patient's perspective. As skillful as a therapist is, it is difficult to assess how closely the patient's observations match reality. For instance, a patient might be saying that a boss is mistreating him, when in fact the boss is acting in a manner typical of bosses, such as pressing the employee to finish a task. Even in a situation in which the therapist meets a potential spouse, her viewpoint has been affected by having heard the patient's observations over an extended time. Patients may also not recognize or communicate their own role in interpersonal conflicts. It is not unusual to learn from another source about problematic behaviors that the patient is not aware of. Although some therapists recommend contact with other people in the patient's life as a source of information, this will not be a focus of the approaches recommended here. Psychodynamic therapists can use their knowledge of how patients' perceptions of others may be distorted based on intrapsychic conflicts and characterological tendencies, but it is important to recognize that this can still lead to misjudgments.

## Countertransference Issues

Therapists' countertransferences can cloud their perspective on patients' circumstances and decision making (Gabbard 2014). Therapists can do their best to be aware of these countertransferences, but they are not always successful in containing them. For instance, a therapist whose father was a demanding authority figure could inappropriately encourage a patient to confront her boss because of rebellious urges or discourage assertion because of excessive fears of confrontation. However, it could be argued that therapists should monitor and modulate their countertransference under any circumstances, and the countertransference risk from addressing behavioral change is no greater than the risk from any other analytic intervention.

Another countertransference factor that can arise is the belief that one knows better than the patient about what to do in various life circumstances. Therapists can develop a somewhat grandiose sense of their capabilities, feeling that they know best. Although therapists may indeed be more capable of negotiating certain problems in relationships, they should acknowledge that they often cannot know what is best for the patient in various circumstances. Additionally, a therapist may become frustrated with a patient's inability or resistance to carrying out a certain task. Therapists might focus on a patient's resistance or even express annoyance as the patient struggles to make particular changes.

The tools that psychoanalysts typically use can be valuable in these circumstances. Therapists should be alert to internal cues that suggest a countertransference problem is occurring, such as feeling they know what is best for patients, insisting the patient take a particular action, or engaging in a power struggle. To the extent that these feelings and behaviors emerge, they may be clues that a patient is resisting therapeutic interventions in a way that the therapist may be struggling with. For instance, the therapist may feel either dismissed or devalued, in covert or overt ways. In some instances, the patient is struggling to address these tasks, but the therapist experiences the patient as resistant.

### Case Example

Ms. F, a 48-year-old divorced nurse with a 16-year-old son, struggled over many years with setting appropriate limits for her child. The problem had been addressed from many different psychodynamic perspectives, attempting to identify why the patient had difficulty maintaining these limits. Ms. F described her own struggles with a mother who was overly critical of her, particularly her weight, and would be very reactive to the patient expressing any needs of her mother's time or concern, either yelling at her or withdrawing. Her mother also had recurrent depressive episodes, and the patient feared that her mother would become even more withdrawn if she expressed a wish for her help or support. Overall, Ms. F came to believe that she needed to yield her needs to others, as well as appease them, to avert rejection or withdrawal.

Ms. F would routinely be upended by her son saying, "You can't tell me what to do." At times the therapist became frustrated by the patient's inability to react with consistent limits. He was aware of his frustration and made efforts not to express it to the patient, although he struggled with avoiding showing these feelings. He recognized that expressing anger toward the patient was only likely to exacerbate her frustration and inhibitions, and that she would feel criticized like she did with her mother. The therapist felt at these times as if Ms. F was not listening to him or was disregarding him. He considered the possibility that Ms. F was demonstrating a resistance to his efforts based on an intrapsychic conflict or a rebellious tendency. Although this was possible, the patient seemed quite attentive and interested in changing, and agreed with the therapist's identification of her problems and the conflicts contributing to them.

He began to recognize that this was likely a dissociative phenomenon, related to the stress the patient felt with her mother:

> Therapist: It seems to me some kind of disconnect must occur when you are in that situation, because I know you understand what to say, but you can't follow up with it.
> Ms. F: I know it's a big problem. I get it but I just don't seem to be able to think about it at that point.
> Th: I wonder if it's because you were so threatened and upset about the problems with your mother that you just feel in the grip of the danger, and become unable to think.
> Ms. F: I mean that sounds like it makes sense. What do I need to do?
> Th: Well, we need to think of some way for you to step back from the situation. Possibly there may be a way of staying connected to me at those points that can allow these other ideas to come into play.
> Ms. F: Okay, well that sounds like a helpful way of thinking about it.

The realization of this likely dissociative tendency helped to ease the therapist's frustration with the patient's difficulties. He recognized how the patient's capacity to mentalize had been disrupted and that efforts should be focused on how to reestablish it.

# A Collaborative Approach to Behavioral Change

In order to reduce the risks of problems deriving from behavioral change efforts, the therapist should identify and encourage collaborative aspects of this process, including sharing the uncertainty of the process. After determining which behaviors are likely problematic, the therapist looks with the patient at formulations for understanding the behavior and at possible behavioral alternatives. Although suggesting a particular course of action, the therapist can acknowledge that he or she cannot know the most effective behavior in a particular circumstance based on the factors described in this chapter. For example, the therapist could advise a patient who routinely allows others to mistreat him to increase his efforts to stop the mistreatment, and explore inhibitions about asserting himself. The therapist can discuss with the patient that there is a risk that being assertive could lead to new difficulties, but there are clear problems in accepting a persistently problematic interpersonal situation. The therapist will help the patient to understand the behavior in relation to the patient's intrapsychic conflicts, developmental influences, and characterological difficulties, and identify issues that interfere with behavioral change. Therapists can encourage patients to raise concerns and feelings about suggested behaviors. A patient's rebellious reaction to collaborative efforts can be examined in the context of feelings about the therapist. In the following vignette, the therapist explored the patient's wary and angry response to developing a collaborative approach to his job search.

### Case Example

Mr. G, a 46-year-old freelance writer, felt angry that he could not find adequately paying assignments and that his talents as a writer were not sufficiently recognized. Others were pressuring him to find any kind of supplemental work, including as an administrative assistant, which he considered demeaning. He was very wary that the therapist would also encourage him to look for one of these jobs. In his treatment with prior therapists he had signaled that he did not want to be "pushed" to get a job like this. He anticipated that the therapist, like many others, would not recognize that he felt unable to tolerate working in a job of this nature. He would refer to this struggle as "I can't" rather than "I won't." He was particularly furious with his wife for pressing him to find any kind of job, even as he acknowledged her concerns about their long-term financial stability. The therapist noted the patient's increasing anger as he attempted to address the struggle with the job search.

> Mr. G: So my wife is really stepping up the pressure on me about the job.
> Therapist: I guess when we discuss the issue about your work it's difficult because you get very frustrated about it.
> Mr. G: Well, that's because I don't think you get it either. I don't think you recognize how I really can't work in these circumstances. It makes me lose interest in it even more.
> Th: Yes, I understand that's the case. When we attempt to look at why you feel it's intolerable to work in these settings you see it as my wanting you to get one of those jobs.
> Mr. G: Well, I guess I hadn't looked at it that way. When I think about it I just feel like I'm undermined and I would feel terrible about myself.
> Th: Well, I think we need to understand more about this. I know you felt that your parents convinced you that you were destined to be very special.
> Mr. G: Yes. That's true. They always thought I would be a great writer from early on for some reason. I guess I showed some

> early talent, and even in fifth grade they sent me to get extra tutoring on my writing. I did win a couple prizes in high school, but I really didn't work on anything else.
>
> Th: It seems like your parents didn't help you to recognize limitations about your skills.
>
> Mr. G: I guess not, but I really feel annoyed that much of my work gets rejected. And if I had to get a regular job I'd feel humiliated. But maybe that's an over-the-top reaction.

The patient believed that any effort to explore his conflicts and feelings about a job search represented an attempt to pressure him to find work he considered menial and intolerable. A transference interpretation helped the patient to realize he inaccurately anticipated this from the therapist, allowing a shift toward a more positive therapeutic alliance and collaborative stance. At that point, the therapist was able to identify developmental factors that contributed to his frustrations with others and his job search.

## References

Busch FN, Milrod BL: Psychodynamic treatment for separation anxiety in a treatment nonresponder. J Am Psychoanal Assoc 63(5):893–919, 2015 26487108

Busch FN, Milrod BL, Singer M, et al: Panic-Focused Psychodynamic Psychotherapy—eXtended Range. New York, Routledge, 2012

Gabbard GO: Psychodynamic assessment of the patient, in Psychodynamic Psychiatry in Clinical Practice, 5th Edition. Washington, DC, American Psychiatric Publishing, 2014, pp 79–97

Thoma N, Pilecki B, McKay D: Contemporary cognitive behavior therapy: a review of theory, history, and evidence. Psychodyn Psychiatry 43(3):423–461, 2015 26301761

# Using Psychodynamic Techniques in Addressing Behavioral Change

This chapter describes traditional psychoanalytic techniques along with modifications of them to aid in behavioral change. These techniques include free association, clarification, and confrontation; interpretation of intrapsychic conflicts, defenses, and the transference; development of mentalization skills; working through; and use of countertransference (Table 4–1). Case examples will demonstrate how these approaches are integrated with targeting behavioral change. Chapter 5 ("A Framework for Targeting Behavioral Change") will provide a framework to target behavioral change per se.

## Free Association

In the technique of free association, the therapist encourages the patient to say whatever comes to mind. The technique is meant to aid patients to not screen their thoughts, feelings, and fantasies, allowing access to mental states that feel conflicted and trigger emotional discomfort. Inherently, patients will screen in spite of this effort, and the therapist should be alert to the patient's hesitation or avoidance of certain mental contents.

**TABLE 4–1.** Psychoanalytic techniques

Free association: encouraging patient to say whatever comes to mind

Clarification and confrontation: identifying patients' typical patterns of thought, feelings, or behavior

Interpretation: linking observed behaviors, emotions, and thoughts to dynamic factors that contribute to them

   Conflict: identifies unconscious wishes or fantasies, emotions that are triggered, and internalized prohibitions

   Defense: identifies ways in which patients characteristically defend themselves from painful affects or conflicted fantasies; examples:

     Passive aggression

     Reaction formation

     Identification with the aggressor

   Genetic (as in genesis): links past experiences, perceptions, or fantasies with current thoughts or behavior

   Transference: identifies feelings and fantasies from prior significant relationships as they emerge with the therapist

Development of mentalization skills

Working through

Use of countertransference

---

In psychodynamic psychotherapy that addresses behavior, the therapist will intervene in the patient's free associational process to make clarifications and interpretations targeting behavioral change and to consider certain alternatives. Nevertheless, this technique remains valuable in accessing mental content that contributes to inhibitions or problematic behaviors. This approach is used, for example, in helping patients to identify what feelings and fantasies are present as they consider enacting particular behaviors, such as "What comes to mind as you think about talking to your husband about wanting him to do more chores?" as described in Chapter 7 ("Identifying Alternative Behaviors").

## Clarification and Confrontation

Clarification and confrontation are techniques in which the therapist points out a patient's typical patterns of thought, feelings, or behavior. Clarifications do not address the patient's unconscious motivations or developmental contributions to these patterns. Rather, they are used to bring attention to problematic thought or behavior patterns or to question a characteristic mode of perception or behavior that adds to the patient's difficulties. Confrontation identifies a pattern of contradictory sets of beliefs, attitudes, or behaviors that the patient appears to be unaware of. Clarification and confrontation aid in the development of the patient's capacity for self-observation by enlisting the observing ego in developing objectivity about the self.

In terms of behavioral change, the core aspect of clarification and confrontation is identifying a problematic behavioral pattern, along with particular affects, fantasies, or conflicts that precede or trigger these behaviors. Examples might include the following: "I notice that when you become frustrated with your wife, you withdraw and avoid her rather than address the problem you are having with her," or "I've observed that when you feel threatened at work, you attack one of your subordinates rather than acknowledge to yourself the problems you are having." A confrontation is illustrated in the following exchange:

> Therapist: I notice you say that you are frustrated with your wife's tendency to depend on you, but then you often continue to take care of her, like organizing her pills and putting them out for her to take.
> Mr. H: Oh, yes. That's true. I think I need to do that. She would screw it up.
> Th: Well, have you attempted to teach her about the pills or observe to see if she can do it herself?
> Mr. H: No, I haven't done that.
> Th: So it makes me wonder sometimes if in fact you like taking care of her or that she needs you, even though at other times you say it frustrates you.
> Mr. H: I would have to think about that. I haven't been aware of it.

## Interpretation

Interpretations link observed behaviors, emotions, and thoughts to the dynamic factors that contribute to them. The therapist develops and shares a hypothesis about specific, typically unconscious, intrapsychic conflicts and defenses that trigger symptoms or problematic behaviors and may connect these patterns to the transference and developmental factors. An effective interpretation can lead to recall of memories, feelings, and fantasies relevant to the patient's current situation and to changes in the patient's themes, symptoms, and behaviors. Interpretations are developed and modified over the course of treatment, providing a growing framework of dynamic factors and interventions relevant to particular symptoms and behaviors. They are elaborated in different contexts in the process of working through, a phase of therapy in which dynamics are explored in greater depth and a broader array of behavioral changes are considered (see below).

There are various subtypes of interpretations, including those focusing on conflicts, defenses, developmental factors, and the transference. A conflict interpretation describes an unconscious wish or fantasy and the internalized prohibitions and emotional reactions that this fantasy triggers, such as guilt or fear. A common example would be identifying a wish to hurt or criticize another person along with anxiety and guilt about harm or damage and fears of retaliation. Therapists may also interpret two wishes that are experienced as contradictory, such as to love and hurt another person. Defense interpretations consider the ways in which patients characteristically defend themselves from painful affects, negative perceptions of themselves and others, or threatening unconscious fantasies, which can include identifying specific defense mechanisms or behaviors. An example of a defense interpretation would be suggesting to a patient that he is frightened of being angry and defends against these feelings by a compensatory submissiveness or taking care of others, as in the case of reaction formation. Interpretations focusing on developmental factors, which have been termed "genetic" (as in genesis), link past experiences, perceptions, or fantasies with current thoughts or behavior. Transference interpretations identify how the experience of the therapist represents perceptions, emotions, and conflicts from prior significant relationships.

The following vignette provides examples of clarification and interpretation in the case of Ms. I, whose case is discussed in greater depth in Chapter 5, with a focus on behavioral change.

### Case Example

Ms. I, a lawyer, struggled with addressing problems with her husband, Tom. An important factor in her background was chronic fighting between her parents and her older sister.

> Ms. I: I can't get Tom to make changes in his behavior, so I just get very demoralized.

Therapist: What are you dealing with right now?

Ms. I: He avoids getting together with other people, and so we can't have social activities. I really want him to do it, but he always has an excuse. A lot of the time he's focused on his physical complaints as an excuse. But I think he's mainly nervous around people.

Th: How do you handle that?

Ms. I: I try to push him to go, but he starts saying, "I don't feel like doing it while I'm recovering from Lyme disease" or "I'm busy looking for a job now. It's hard to make plans."

Th: What do you feel then?

Ms. I: I get anxious. I don't want to hurt him; if I push him he may feel badly about his fears of people or his health. When I say he might be worried he says, "I don't have social anxiety. I have friends but they don't live around here." And that's when I start to feel demoralized and frightened.

Th: I know you're concerned about hurting him, but you also think he should get checked out by a doctor to see what's going on with his health. What frightens you about encouraging him more?

Ms. I: I think back to my sister and father fighting. And I see this look on my father's face of just feeling hurt and demoralized after my sister cursed at him. And I think Tom will feel the same way. And then he may lash out like my father, when he yelled at my sister in response to her attacking him.

Th: So you feel as if you're in that situation, even though the circumstances with your husband are quite different, and therefore any expression of frustration feels dangerous, potentially explosive and damaging.

Ms. I: Well, I wasn't even thinking I felt frustrated at that point, but it makes sense that I do.

This vignette includes clarification of a pattern, as well as the interpretation of a conflict that led the patient to struggle with being assertive with her husband: Ms. I believed that any comments about problems in a relationship may be explosive and damaging to the other person. Internally she had a wish to express her anger at her husband, such as by screaming at him, just as she wished she could at her fighting family members. However, she felt guilty and fearful about the potential damage her anger could inflict or inciting anger in the other person. Shortly after the identification of this pattern, her increased safety with angry feelings allowed her to more directly challenge her husband's stance, though she still struggled.

Ms. I: I wanted to go out this weekend, but he said could we wait until next weekend because he thought he'd be feeling better. And this time I noticed I got angry instead of anxious.
Th: How did you handle it?
Ms. I: Well, I got very worried for a moment. But then I settled down, and I said, "Look, Tom. It's important for me to go out. And I want you to compromise." And then he agreed to do it.
Th: So identifying that you're angry in those circumstances is a really important step.
Ms. I: Yes, but you know, I'm still worried about it. It feels very intense. And I feel I struggle to control it.
Th: Now that you have access to feeling angry you have the opportunity to better understand and manage it. You also found out that rather than damaging him it seemed to help him feel less anxious and the two of you to feel better about your relationship.

## Addressing Defenses

Defense mechanisms represent characteristic modes of managing conflicted or frightening feelings and fantasies, typically operating at an unconscious level (see Busch et al. 2016). Defensive avoidance of intolerable or frightening emotions or thoughts, such as angry thoughts and feelings, will interfere with access to emotional information that is necessary to properly address problematic behaviors. Identifying and interpreting the use of these defenses aids in accessing the warded off feelings and fantasies. Although a variety of defenses can contribute to behavioral problems, the defenses of passive aggression, reaction formation, and identification with the aggressor are particularly important.

### *Passive Aggression*

Passive aggression is a defense mechanism in which anger is denied or minimized and expressed indirectly through passive behaviors, such as lateness or "forgetting" an appointment. This mechanism averts an unconscious threat associated with more overt expressions of aggression. However, these behaviors are problematic in that rather than express grievances in a productive manner, patients inadvertently provoke others' frustration. As they are typically unaware of the behavior, patients often have trouble comprehending others' anger toward them in response to passive aggression. An important goal of psychodynamic psychotherapy targeting behavior is helping patients to recognize this defense and to identify the various fantasies and conflicts that interfere with a more direct and effective expression of angry feelings. Included in this exploration is determining what is triggering patients' frustration to better address the sources of their distress.

## Case Example

Mr. J, a 56-year-old married accountant with dysthymia, was very frustrated with his wife. He felt that she had not responded to him sexually early in their marriage and that, despite renewed sexual interest, did not view him with any passion. Mr. J described withholding sex from his wife and did not perform professionally as she hoped he would, seemingly on a long-standing quest to retaliate against her. The patient had difficulty admitting that these behaviors were intended as revenge.

> Mr. J: When we went into the marriage, I wanted to have sex with her, and she wasn't responsive to me. So why would I want to respond to her needs now?
> Therapist: It sounds as if you're trying to get back at her.
> Mr. J: Well, I guess I am, in a way. I don't usually think of it like that. I really think of myself as a nice guy.
> Th: Does she know about your frustrations with her?
> Mr. J: Not really. I mean, she's frustrated about my not responding to her sexually, but I haven't really told her why. I mean, what you're calling the revenge thing.
> Th: Why not?
> Mr. J: I don't really want to hurt her feelings. I think it would make her feel really bad.
> Th: But it sounds like that's the net effect of your withholding sexually anyway.
> Mr. J: Yes. I guess so.

Through these clarifications, Mr. J was ultimately able to see that his behavior toward his wife was vengeful, even though he expressed it in a passive, withholding manner. A major problem with Mr. J's approach was that his own feelings of inadequacy were heightened by his not dealing more effectively with his wife. In fact, he blocked his own professional success, which he felt badly about and which further alienated his wife, causing her to be even less supportive. Identifying his passive aggressive defenses helped Mr. J to more directly address his frustrations with her.

## Reaction Formation

When using the defense mechanism of reaction formation, patients disavow frightening or conflicted feelings by unconsciously converting them to their opposites. The most common problematic expression of this defense is anger being changed into a positive or helpful feeling, but intolerable loving emotions may also shift to consciously experienced anger. As with passive aggression, reaction formation leads to problematic behavior because patients cannot access negative feelings necessary to express frustration about issues that cause distress. The therapist can identify the use of reaction formation when patients express positive feelings toward someone with whom they are at odds or having problems. The therapist can suggest the patients are having difficulty accessing underlying anger and its triggers.

### Case Example

Ms. K, a 24-year-old public relations consultant, became involved with Bob, who was quite needful of her support because he was depressed about losing his job and having financial woes. She expressed significant concerns about the relationship because she had a pattern of becoming involved with men who were dependent on her and then becoming frustrated and disappointed with them. When the therapist explored what attracted the patient to Bob in spite of his problems, Ms. K focused on her boyfriend's positive traits, including his intelligence, congeniality, and warmth.

Over time, however, the boyfriend's dependency intensified. He moved in with the patient because of his financial difficulties and spent much of his time "hanging out" at her apartment, doing little in the way of housework. Ms. K began to get increasingly depressed. She felt exhausted by Bob's problems, even though she felt she still needed to help him. She also became very self-critical about her tendency to get involved with needy men. However, she expressed little direct anger toward him.

> Therapist: It seems like you would be more frustrated with Bob! It sounds as if he's really not doing much to earn his keep.
> Ms. K: He just really needs help. The problem's mine for getting involved with guys like this. I've got to try to understand more about that.
> Th: I certainly agree with you, but how do you feel about how he's conducting his life at this point?
> Ms. K: Well, I guess he could be doing more to help out me and himself. He's not looking for a job, but he could at least clean up the dishes. I mean, I'm supporting him.
> Th: Have you spoken to him about this?
> Ms. K: Well, some. But I don't want to get him even more upset. He really feels bad about himself.

Further exploration of the patient's pull toward needy men proved to be of value, allowing a genetic interpretation that further aided the patient's insight. Ms. K's father was distant and critical, a successful entrepreneur who showed little emotion. She described her mother, on the other hand, as emotionally more connected to her, although acknowledging that she was also rather self-involved and somewhat depressed. Ms. K believed that when she was needed by others, her attachment would be closer and more intimate. She feared getting angry because she worried that the man might be "sensitive" like her mother and feel injured, disrupting their tie. However, she became demoralized when she felt she was not getting what she needed from her relationships, including sexually.

As therapeutic work on this issue continued, Ms. K became increasingly aware of her frustration. She then decided that she needed to take some action, so she pressed her boyfriend to get a job and find his own place. To her surprise, he responded positively to these suggestions. As he became more independent, their satisfaction with the relationship increased.

This interpretation demonstrates how access to underlying angry feelings that are being defended against can aid behavioral change.

## Identification With the Aggressor

In the defense of identification with the aggressor, patients link their self-image with someone whom they experienced or fantasized as having power and dominance, particularly someone with whom they were vulnerable in the past. Patients may unconsciously use this defense mechanism to combat feelings of inadequacy and gain a sense of being empowered and in control. However, this stance often causes guilty feelings, particularly about wishes to dominate or hurt others in the ways that they had previously felt bullied or threatened. This defense mechanism often interferes with assertive behaviors, as patients can confuse their normal assertion with wishes and actions that they perceive as damaging.

### Case Example

Mr. L, a 52-year-old lawyer with chronic depression, had significant difficulty pressing his staff members to complete their tasks properly, as he wanted to be seen as a friend rather than a boss. He accepted weak excuses for their need to leave early or take days off and was very accepting of shoddy work. However, he would obsess angrily about his employees not adequately doing their job and blamed them in part for the limited success of his practice. Occasionally he would mildly reproach one of them and was frustrated that he seemed unable to get others to follow his rules.

> Therapist: Why do you think you have difficulty making more demands on your employees?
> Mr. L: Well, I'm scared they'll quit, and then I'll be stuck training a new person. I also want to be seen as the good guy. I don't want to hurt their feelings.
> Th: What do you mean by that?
> Mr. L: I feel that if I criticize them, I'll get really nasty or abusive and just make them feel very badly.
> Th: I think it's important for us to understand more about this, especially as you don't give any indication you would actually behave that way.

Mr. L's background again proved relevant to this issue, describing his parents as very unfair and rigid about rules. He was often upbraided about minor infractions (coming home a few minutes late for curfew) or for not making better grades, even though he found school difficult. He was furious with his parents, but if he got angry directly, his mother would "withdraw her love" and not speak to him for days. This caused him great anguish, and he struggled between his wish to be a "good boy" and his anger at what he regarded as unfair treatment. The therapist discussed with Mr. L how viewing himself as an assertive boss was identified in his mind with his parents' criticisms of him, an example of identification with the aggressor.

> Th: It's interesting that when you describe what you're worried you would do as a boss critiquing your employees, your behavior sounds just like your parents with you.
> Mr. L: Yes. I guess it does. I mean, I don't want to be unfair and to hurt people the way they did with me. I know what it feels like.
> Th: It sounds as if you really feel guilty when you need to critique your employees, even though you actually tend to be overly polite.
> Mr. L: Yeah. I've always worried that if I really allowed myself more power, I'd walk all over everybody.
> Th: I think we need to help you more with this feeling, particularly because it is so inhibiting and your behavior is so clearly at odds with your fears.

Here, again, an important goal, in addition to self-understanding, is to aid the patient in changing his behavior, allowing him to set better limits with his employees. To this end, the therapist had to detoxify the dangers Mr. L associated with being the authority.

## Working With Transference

In the transference (Freud 1905[1901]/1953), the patient experiences emotions and perceptions of prior significant relationships with the therapist, allowing for exploration and identification of fantasies and conflicts. Interpreting the transference enables patients to understand characteristic ways in which they misperceive others, and these observations usually generalize to other important relationships (Cooper 1987; Westen and Gabbard 2002). These interpretations help patients to develop an increased awareness of their motivations and actions, giving them more information to shift behaviors. Feelings and conflicts regarding the therapist can also help to identify specific triggers of problematic behaviors, such as patients becoming withdrawn when angry feelings and fantasies about the therapist emerge. The therapist's nonjudgmental stance in response to patients' feelings is crucial in providing a sense of safety for unconscious fantasies to emerge, as patients typically anticipate a negative or perhaps intrusive response.

Some patients readily express their feelings and fantasies about the therapist, allowing for early interpretations of the transference, whereas others are more reticent. The therapist should stay alert for indications of the patient's reactions to her and call attention to them when appropriate. Failure to identify the transference may intensify patients' fears that the therapist cannot tolerate certain feelings, just as they often experienced with their caregivers. Alternatively, early, aggressive focus by the therapist on the transference can be experienced as intrusive, potentially triggering denial and anger. If a patient becomes angry or anxious when his feelings about the therapist are identified, this reaction should also be addressed. This intervention can lead to valuable insights about the patient's conflicts and discomfort with examining the transference, and can be linked to problems with other relationships. Another opportunity for transference interpretation occurs when an otherwise positive therapeutic alliance becomes disrupted (Safran and Muran 2000), allowing for exploration of what led to the tensions. Whenever the therapeutic work stalls, the therapist should consider feelings and fantasies about the therapist as a potential source. Examples of transference reactions will be provided in the two central cases in Chapter 5.

On occasion, patients will demonstrate certain problematic behaviors within the treatment, referred to as *enactments*. For instance, passive aggressive enactments can include arriving late to appointments or late payment of bills. Patients may miss or "forget" a session after discussing a difficult topic or avoid raising a topic that they are frustrated about, such as occurred with Mr. C in Chapter 3 ("Identifying and Addressing Risks in Targeting Behavioral Change"). These enactments provide opportunities to examine behavioral problems in the context of the transference relationship, with more direct access to triggering cues, feelings, and conflicts in a nonjudgmental setting. The therapist should be aware, however, that patients may experience examining these behaviors as threatening, because they are wary of the fantasies and feelings that may emerge with the therapist.

# Development of Mentalization Skills

Therapists help patients develop mentalization skills by encouraging them to consider what is going on in their own minds as well as the minds of others. At times the therapist may suggest motives for someone else's behavior to model mentalizing skills.

### Case Example

A 42-year-old man who worked in public relations, Mr. M, expressed frustration about his husband's behavior:

> Mr. M: I just don't get why he goes out every night. I'm not even sure he loves me anymore
> Therapist: Why do you think he might be doing that?
> Mr. M: I don't know. I just like to sit at home and read. I guess we just like different activities. But I don't get why he's doing it even more.
> Th: Well I'm thinking that last week you told me that he was very angry about your drinking. Do you think that could have anything to do with it.
> Mr. M: Well I guess it could be. I hadn't really connected those things.
> Th: Well you had said that he complained about feeling alone when you were drinking and reading. Maybe he's feeling rejected by you.
> Mr. M: That's possible. I've tried to cut back my drinking but it's difficult. Partly because I'm mad and lonely.

> Th: Well it sounds like you might be caught in a vicious cycle with him. Maybe you two should try going out together to something you both enjoy. And probably something that doesn't involve drinking.
>
> Mr. M: Yeah. Well it might be hard to find an activity we both like but I'll talk to him.

This work on mentalization helped the patient to understand his perception of being rejected and to identify behavioral changes that might be helpful to his relationship. Over time most patients will learn to employ these mentalization skills.

## Working Through

Working through involves the process of identifying various dynamic contributors to symptoms and behavioral problems and how they emerge in different contexts and circumstances. This process is particularly important in addressing behavioral problems, which tend to persist in part because of the multiple contributing factors and functions that they serve. For instance, patients may fear assertiveness because of frightening responses from caregivers to assertive behaviors during childhood; harbor fantasies of damaging others through self-assertion; experience fear of losing an attachment to important others; and/or have guilt about wishes to harm, control, or humiliate others linked unconsciously with assertive behaviors. These dynamics can emerge and affect behavior in a variety of contexts, including with partners, bosses, and friends. Over the course of treatment, the patient develops an increased awareness and understanding of these dynamics, examining them in a variety of circumstances, providing increased opportunities and strategies to intervene with the behavior. For instance, patients may need to become aware of anger that is denied, tolerate and accept anger, identify triggers of these feelings, and learn to express anger appropriately. Several examples of working through are provided in this book.

## Use of Countertransference

Clinicians should always scan their feelings, fantasies, and reactions to patients, as the therapist can use this information to avoid enacting problematic countertransference reactions and to identify certain experiences of the patient. These feelings and fantasies can also be an indication of the presence of significant and meaningful transference. Once clinicians become aware of these feelings, they should carefully evaluate the clinical material for what they are responding to in the patients' verbal and nonverbal behavior. Clinicians should consider to what degree they are reacting to particular issues of patients and/or are having emotional responses to certain experiences based on their own dynamics (Gabbard 1995; Searles 1959). It is generally recommended that dynamic therapists have their own treatment during their training to better understand their intrapsychic conflicts and to identify areas of vulnerability to countertransference. An example of countertransference was provided in the case of Ms. F in Chapter 3.

## References

Busch FN, Rudden MG, Shapiro T: Psychodynamic Treatment of Depression, 2nd Edition. Arlington, VA, American Psychiatric Publishing, 2016

Cooper AM: Changes in psychoanalytic ideas: transference interpretation. J Am Psychoanal Assoc 35(1):77–98, 1987 3584822

Freud S: Fragment of an analysis of a case of hysteria (1905[1901]), in Standard Edition of the Complete Psychological Works of Sigmund Freud, Vol 7. Translated and edited by Strachey J. London, Hogarth Press, 1953, pp 1–122

Gabbard GO: Countertransference: the emerging common ground. Int J Psychoanal 76(Pt 3):475–485, 1995 7558607

Safran JD, Muran JC: Negotiating the Therapeutic Alliance. New York, Guilford, 2000

Searles HF: Oedipal love in the countertransference. Int J Psychoanal 40:180–190, 1959 14444362

Westen D, Gabbard GO: Developments in cognitive neuroscience: II. Implications for theories of transference. J Am Psychoanal Assoc 50(1):99–134, 2002 12018876

# 5

# A Framework for Targeting Behavioral Change

**A** framework will be described for understanding and formulating behavioral problems, identifying alternative behaviors, addressing interfering factors, and monitoring the impact of behavioral change (Table 5–1). The potential use of homework in targeting behavioral change will also be discussed. These approaches represent a significant shift from more traditional psychodynamic psychotherapies and are described in greater depth in the chapters that follow (Chapters 6 through 9). Assertiveness and anger will be used as key areas of behavioral inhibition or expression to provide examples and illustrate this framework and associated techniques. As noted in Chapter 2 ("Understanding Psychodynamic Factors That Impede Behavioral Change"), patients with a variety of symptom complexes and personality disorders often struggle with attaining an appropriate degree of assertiveness or the effective expression of anger (Busch et al. 2012, 2016). The framework begins with identifying behavioral problems, a process that occurs in conjunction with the formulation of dynamic contributors to these difficulties.

**TABLE 5–1.** Targeting behavioral change

Determining whether behaviors are problematic
Identifying problematic behaviors
Examining the context, affects, and meanings of problematic behaviors
Arriving at a formulation of contributing intrapsychic conflicts, defenses, and developmental factors
Identifying alternative behaviors
Elaborating feelings and fantasies about performing alternative behaviors
Addressing factors that interfere with alternative behaviors
Working with the impact of behavioral change
Making use of homework

## Determining Whether Behaviors Are Problematic

How does one determine if a behavior is problematic? And how can the therapist or patient ensure that a change in behavior is adequate or effectively expressed? Inherently, a behavioral pattern is viewed as problematic to the degree that it creates difficulties for the patient, and the patient has little flexibility in varying the behavior in the contexts in which it leads to problems. Patients may or may not recognize that a behavior is causing them difficulties, and certain problematic behaviors may be called to their attention by others. They may be conflicted about recognizing that a behavior causes trouble, especially if there is a partial adaptive or defensive purpose to it. Work at identifying and changing problematic behaviors continues over the course of a psychotherapeutic treatment.

Inhibitions or expressions of assertiveness or anger occur in several problematic ways. Individuals may demonstrate an overall inhibition in assertion or excessive expressions of anger. They may shift between overly inhibited and overly aggressive behavior. They may have difficulty adjusting their assertiveness and anger as required by different circumstances. These various manifestations often have adverse effects on patients' relationships.

The psychodynamic formulation of difficulties with assertiveness includes core conflicts involving fears that others may be damaged, rejecting, or critical in response to these behaviors (see Chapter 2). These expectations can derive in part from actual problematic responses from caregivers and others to assertive behaviors during development that have become internalized as self and object representations and unconscious fantasies (Busch et al. 2012). An unconscious (and sometimes conscious) link between assertiveness and angry competitive feelings and fantasies can intensify fears of hurting others and anticipated retaliation, triggering guilt with anger being directed toward the self. The following brief vignette provides an instance of identifying relevant dynamics, which were employed to recognize and address problematic behaviors.

### Case Example

Mr. N, a 54-year-old accountant, who suffered from panic disorder, struggled with his father's demands on him, even though his father was elderly and somewhat debilitated. These dictates included a series of directives regarding the care of his father's apartment and expecting the patient to be present for chores even when it problematically disrupted his own life and work. His father was also refusing to get a home care attendant, even though his doctors had warned him against living on his own. The therapist and patient identified his inability to say no to his father as a problem, given his incapacity to be flexible in his response and the difficulties his compliance was creating for him.

On exploration, Mr. N described a lifetime of feeling bullied or undermined by his father. He experienced panic attacks in the context of dealing with bullying clients pressuring him to do things that he did not believe were ethical. It emerged in the course of exploration that Mr. N was enraged with his father and clients and had guilty fantasies of being physically violent toward or bullying them. As these fantasies were explored, and he began to feel safer with these feelings and urges, his anxiety and guilt diminished. Various behavioral alternatives had been discussed when he told his father he would not help him if he refused to get a home care attendant. To his surprise his father, rather than reacting angrily, quickly accepted this arrangement.

Two more extended cases are now presented to demonstrate the use of specific behavior targeting techniques in psychodynamic psychotherapy. The patients in these cases primarily experienced inhibitions in assertiveness. Cases in which patients excessively express angry impulses and actions will be presented in Chapter 10 ("Engaging the Patient in Addressing Specific Behavioral Problems").

## Case Example

Ms. I, a 44-year-old married partner at a law firm (see Chapter 4), experienced chronic anxiety that would sometimes take the form of somatic preoccupations. In her personal life and work she suffered from wide-ranging problems with assertiveness and tended to become involved in or develop relationships in which she did not assert her own needs and focused on taking care of others. Although she expressed frustration about these relationships, she was highly ambivalent about them, feeling some pleasure from her caretaking, and did not believe she could do anything to change these circumstances. She experienced any attempt to confront other individuals as potentially damaging to them or causing them to reject her, and therefore rarely made this effort.

Her husband, Tom, was unemployed for long stretches, and his motivation to work was limited. He suffered from a variety of somatic symptoms that affected his energy and concentration, although the medical cause was unclear and he was unwilling to see a doctor. Ms. I alternated between feeling furious and sorry for him, and a guilty concern about her anger. In addition to earning the income in the family, she would typically prepare dinner and clean up. She acknowledged experiencing him to some degree as a child to be cared for, and in this way he acted indirectly as a replacement for her not having had children. In addition to the caretaking he required, he tended to be controlling, wanting to limit her social activity. On occasion she would become aware of her frustration but feared expressing it toward him, either by pressing him to find a job, see a doctor, or stop his controlling behavior. Such a confrontation, she believed, would damage him by worsening his insecurity or cause him to be furious with her and withdraw emotionally. She experienced similar problems at her job, in which she had difficulties with holding her associates to deadlines. In many instances she would end up doing their work. As with her husband she feared confronting them about their inadequate efforts, believing that they would feel humiliated by her comments.

Ms. I described the focal point of her early family relationships as intense conflict involving her parents and rebellious older sister, from the time the patient was 10 years old. Ms. I came to fear the frequent explosive arguments in her teen years that took place as her parents, particularly her father, attempted to set limits with her sister or confront her about disrespectful behavior. She alternated between viewing her father as overly tough or harsh toward her sister and thinking that he was easily humiliated, stressed, or overwhelmed in dealing with her. She would keep herself in the background of the arguments, being the "good girl," attempting to help with chores around the home and taking care of her younger brother. She did not want to add any spark to potential conflicts by expressing her own needs or opinions, or trouble her already burdened parents.

## Case Example

Mr. O[1] was a 62-year-old married man who presented with significant depression, including vegetative symptoms. His primary depressive feelings and beliefs centered around a sense of inadequacy. He reported that he no longer felt as effective as he had been at work as a salesman, an important source of self-esteem, as he had lost clients and connections as he grew older. His greatest source of distress was his wife, about 20 years younger than he, whom he felt to be withdrawn and less interested in him sexually. He was worried she might be having an affair, but to some degree he felt that he deserved this, as "I'm not the man I used to be." Mr. O's depressive symptoms responded fairly well to sertraline, but his struggles with self-esteem and assertiveness persisted.

Mr. O described growing up in a family dominated by conflicts with his older brother, who had academic difficulties and a propensity to get into fights both at home and at school. He was fearful of his brother's bullying behavior and the disruptions caused in the family by these conflicts. Nevertheless, the brother was believed to have more business potential and worked in the father's business from early on. Mr. O was pressured to be the good boy, to not create problems, and to yield to his parents' requests. These included doing well at school and complimenting his mother about her clothing or attractiveness. He often felt ignored when the focus was on his brother. His success in his profession in part felt like a way to demonstrate how his parents were wrong about his abilities. His brother struggled professionally, and he acknowledged some guilty pleasure about this. He had left his first wife, whom his mother had wanted him to marry, for a younger woman, his current wife.

Mr. O was unwilling to address his concerns about his wife directly. He denied any anger at her about lack of sexual involvement, but his dreams and fantasies suggested otherwise, including the emergence of information that he was going to masseuses for sexual satisfaction. Exploration revealed that if his wife were having an affair, he would view it as appropriate punishment for leaving his first wife for her. As he increasingly acknowledged anger at his wife, his inhibition about addressing his concerns with her became more evident. He also struggled at work, where he was not being as aggressive as he could be to get sales, and he expressed some guilt about his competitive wishes with coworkers.

# Identifying Behavioral Problems

These patients' primary behavioral problems involved areas of inhibition and unassertiveness, and yielding of their needs to others. They both ac-

---

[1]See Busch et al. 2016.

knowledged these difficulties but at other points appeared to accept these behaviors as understandable based on their fears. It was therefore important to clarify and consistently address these problems, including in each case the patient's justification of them. Ms. I demonstrated an inability to assert herself with her husband with regard to his pursuing employment, seeing a doctor, sharing chores, and limiting their social activity. In addition, she was unable to address problems with her employees, including critiquing their work and setting expectations. Mr. O could not confront his wife about her withdrawn behavior and struggled with being assertive at work, including difficulties competing for sales opportunities.

## Examining the Context, Affects, and Meanings of Problematic Behavior

In order to more effectively address the contributors to problematic behavior and the impediments to change, it is important to identify the context, emotions, and meanings of these actions (see Chapter 6, "Identifying Dynamic Contributors to Problematic Behaviors"). Such efforts occur in therapy sessions along with encouraging patients to observe what they experience at the time of the behavior. These approaches aid patients in developing self-observational capacities and mentalizing skills.

When these factors were explored in therapy, Ms. I's inhibitions were found to intensify in the context of experiencing and expressing frustration toward her husband and her associates at the firm. She believed her efforts to address problems would be overly harsh and damaging, triggering guilt, and feared her assertiveness would lead to her husband's emotional withdrawal. Mr. O became inhibited when he considered confronting his wife, worrying he would upset her, and when competing with his associates. He experienced feelings of inadequacy because of his age, and guilty feelings about past behavior.

## Arriving at a Psychodynamic Formulation of Intrapsychic Conflicts, Defenses, and Developmental Factors That Contribute to Problematic Behavior

As with symptoms, a psychodynamic formulation provides a framework for understanding behavioral difficulties and identifying possible interventions (see Chapter 6). In each of these cases, these patients felt guilty about angry feelings and their needs, and punished themselves through self-criticism and yielding to problematic and hurtful situations. Denial, identification with the aggressor, and reaction formation were prominent defenses. Developmental factors provided important understandings of the origins of these conflicts and behaviors.

Ms. I at first denied angry feelings and fantasies, and when they emerged, she felt guilty for having them and feared they would cause significant damage if expressed. After Ms. I gained more access to her feelings, her anger at times was intense, describing her husband as a "loser" along with thoughts of leaving him. When enraged, she identified with her father and sister as mean and hurtful, an example of identification with the aggressor. She would equate the hurt and humiliated other person to her father, when overwhelmed by her sister's attacks. Her conflicts triggered reaction formation, with increased efforts to care for those she feared harming. Although this defense was initially relieving, she would end up feeling more infuriated about "needing to do everything."

Mr. O needed to deny anger at his wife out of concerns about its intensity and to be the "good boy." He came to recognize that his sexual massages were a passive-aggressive means of getting back at her. He believed he was being punished for leaving his first wife for this younger woman and for competitive wishes toward his brother.

## Identifying Alternative Behaviors

To pursue behavioral change, it is important to identify behavioral alternatives as a potential goal of treatment. Working with patients to consider these alternatives is a significant departure from traditional psychoanalytic technique (see Chapter 7, "Identifying Alternative Behaviors").

Over time, the therapist and Ms. I identified that she could more directly express to her husband the importance of his working and seeing a doctor, and set limits on his restricting her social activity. At her job she could more clearly communicate to her associates about problems meeting their deadlines and ways of improving their work, while reducing her willingness to complete their projects. The therapist and Mr. O determined that he could directly address frustration with his wife about her withdrawal and increase his efforts to compete at obtaining sales.

## Elaborating Feelings and Fantasies About Performing Alternative Behaviors

Once identified, the therapist and patients can explore feelings and conflicts that emerge when alternative behaviors are contemplated. In this approach, the therapist asks patients to imagine performing these behaviors and then consider what their concerns are and what they anticipate as responses from others. Although fears of damage or punishment often arise, more positive feelings, such as excitement and relief about expressing something directly to the other person, can also emerge.

When considering expressing anger or asserting herself in specific situations, Ms. I felt anxious and guilty and believed the other person would be humiliated, irritated, or rejecting. As he considered specific ways of confronting his wife, Mr. O felt guilty about expressing his anger and expected she would be hurt by it or become disinterested or angry, and possibly leave him. As he thought about specific ways of competing for new sales, he anticipated antagonism from his colleagues.

## Addressing Interfering Factors

The therapist develops a framework and strategies for addressing factors that inhibit behavioral changes based on the psychodynamic formulation and fears and fantasies that emerge when considering performing alternative behaviors. Developmental events, intrapsychic conflicts, defenses, self and object representations, transference factors, and mentalization deficits are among the factors that are attended to. The following section demonstrates how the formulation was employed in the cases of Ms. I and Mr. O.

> ### Case Example: Ms. I (*continued*)
> The therapist addressed catastrophic concerns and guilt associated with Ms. I's contemplation of expressing anger and asserting herself. He also examined her need to take care of others to atone for angry feelings and reduce feelings of loss.
>
> Several interventions were aimed at diminishing Ms. I's inhibitions and caretaking efforts and increasing her assertive behavior. These approaches included differentiating her current situation from the apparently out of control circumstances in her childhood home. She and the therapist discussed how her anger or criticisms would almost certainly not damage or humiliate others in the way she anticipated, and she was

very unlikely to express them in the harsh way her sister and parents did. The therapist suggested that communicating heightened expectations to her husband and employees could ultimately aid, rather than harm, their self-esteem by increasing their competence and independence.

The therapist worked to help her recognize and learn to tolerate feelings of loss in her caretaking wishes upon promoting her employees' and husband's efforts at independence. She experienced sadness, including about not having had children, but ultimately felt less frustrated, overwhelmed, and despairing. In addition, the therapist helped her to identify the defense of reaction formation, to recognize that when she felt angry she would shift to extra caretaking to relieve her guilt or unconsciously punish herself.

The following vignettes present some examples of the therapist working with Ms. I to address these factors.

> Ms. I: I find that when I give an associate a directive and they argue with me, that I'll back off and let them do it the way they want, but then later there will be a problem with the work. I said to John, "You need to document what you are doing," and he said, "No I don't." And then I think maybe I'm wrong, so I step back and think I'll let him discover that it doesn't work. But then I end up fixing the problem and he doesn't learn what's necessary.
>
> Therapist: What is your concern in being more direct about what's needed?
>
> Ms. I: That I'll be seen as too controlling and he'll get mad.
>
> Th: This ends up creating a lot of work for you, and you feel more burdened. But I think you back off because you are so frightened of causing hurt or creating a conflict that you need to question yourself and see yourself as incapable. Can you say more about how you imagine John will react?
>
> Ms. I: Well, I do think he would get mad, but when I think about it now I imagine him feeling terribly hurt. I see him making a painful face and feeling devastated. As you've mentioned, this does remind me a bit of my father when he seemed so upset about my sister.
>
> Th: You have said you start to panic when thinking of giving your employee a suggestion. It's as if you were conditioned to fear that any criticism would cause an explosion or hurt on the level of what occurred in your home. Therefore you can't differentiate situations where it may cause some distress but also be quite helpful. You can't gauge the safety of a particular situation because you assume they are all going to lead to danger.

Ms. I: Yes, but I still think he'll be hurt.
Th: I think you fear he will react like your father, but I wonder how likely it is that your associate would be so hurt or angry about your telling him the right way to complete a task. I mean you are his boss. And if he does react like that, the response is a problem, because bosses need to give feedback and instruction to their employees.
Ms. I: I see what you're saying, but it's very tough for me.
Th: Yes, because you feel the other person is too vulnerable to hear your thoughts or needs. But often it doesn't help them or you to keep your thoughts to yourself.
Ms. I: It's true. The other day I did tell John, "Look you have to go back and work on this more," and gave him some instructions for finishing it. He seemed a bit upset but then went and completed the work. It seems like we both felt better.

As she felt safer with her angry feelings, Ms. I increasingly made efforts to confront her husband about her problems with him. However, she struggled at times with a guilty backlash after she made these efforts.

Ms. I: So I told him I was going to go out with my friends despite his foot pain. He said, "Are you sure you want to go out? You seem tired." I got so frustrated I didn't know what to say. I know he was really just thinking about himself.
Th: I guess you could say something about how you appreciate his concern, but perhaps it has more to do with his own worries about not having you there.
Ms. I: That's a good idea. After that he asked, "What will I do for dinner?" Then I started to get hopeless again about changing things. I just said I would make something for him.
Th: It seems when you assert yourself you readily go back to the old place where you feel stuck and helpless, even as you made progress by saying you were going out! I think you feel guilty again that your assertiveness and anger are going to hurt him, and he seems to be implying it will. I think it's certainly worth a discussion that he should be able to figure out what he can do for dinner. It's not as if he can't walk at all, and if need be he could order out! Let's talk about how you might address that with him, and perhaps we can identify more where you get stuck.
Ms. I: Well, I do think when I make the effort and he resists so much I get even more furious with him. Then I get worried. I feel badly for him.

Th: After you make progress and he resists, you get so angry and fearful about damaging him that you need to shut down, and see yourself as weak. I think that you need to make a note that sometimes he will resist your efforts. How else can you handle your anger and guilt at that point, besides giving in on something else?

Ms. I: I think that would be good to work on. I want to keep moving forward.

Although her improvement in assertiveness continued, after a difficult week of struggles at work and home she reported feeling cut off and depressed with a lack of capacity to address her frustrations. She had returned to a focus on her body with cancer fears and feelings of tiredness. She was very angry at Tom, who was considering cutting back his hours at work, and she was fearful he would lose another job. She felt furious at him but was anxious about confronting him. After noting that she was still mad at her associates, she revealed that her husband was pushing her to stop therapy, citing lack of progress, but also because he struggled with her growing assertiveness.

Noting that the patient seemed frustrated about therapy, the therapist believed these circumstances presented an opportunity to explore her conflicts within the transference. He asked if she was also feeling frustrated with the therapy. She hesitantly responded yes and explained that she was "kept" in a previous therapy even when she was not being helped. She did acknowledge that she had made progress in her current treatment.

The therapist encouraged her to express her concerns and irritation about therapy because based on her patterns, she would likely become angry at him but not feel safe expressing it. In fact, because she was frightened about raising these feelings, she tended to ascribe them to someone else, in this case to her husband, who felt somewhat threatened by therapy. She was viewing therapy as a struggle between her needs and the therapist's, in which she would yield to his needs. She was fearful that if she wanted to stop therapy, the therapist would not permit a discussion about goals and length of treatment.

Ms. I was very relieved by the therapist's response, finding him open to her concerns about the treatment. She shifted her tone, and smiling, described several areas of improvement, despite having a difficult week. She acknowledged that based on her fears she brought up her complaint about therapy as if it were her husband's, just as she would tell Tom that her therapist thought his behavior was the problem. The exchange greatly aided Ms. I in increasing her feelings of safety with assertiveness and an understanding of situations where she still felt stuck.

### Case Example: Mr. O (continued)

The therapist worked to increase Mr. O's awareness, acceptance, and tolerance of his anger at his wife. Developmental origins of his pressure to yield to others and fears of expressing frustration were identified. The therapist addressed the patient's guilt and expectation of punishment for leaving his first wife and his competitive wishes. Throughout treatment they considered how he might directly address his wife's withdrawal. As behavioral alternatives were identified, therapist and patient explored what he felt when he imagined confronting her. These factors included fear and guilt about potentially hurting or angering her and underlying feelings of inadequacy.

As treatment progressed, further history emerged about Mr. O's feelings toward his mother, shedding additional light on his guilty reactions. He felt angry at his mother for having pressured him to be the "good boy" and marry his first wife, and he anticipated punishment for these feelings. He had several dreams that symbolized being punished via castration or disempowerment, including one in which he learned his left hand would have to be amputated. The doctor in the dream said to him, underscoring his fantasies, "Well, you're old. You won't be needing it anymore." In a sense, castration as a form of punishment was already occurring in his accepting a lack of sexual activity with his wife. He also felt disempowered in the work setting, believing his colleagues were getting perks he had once received regularly. His fantasies indicated that he experienced his reduced sales as a punishment and that his guilt was inhibiting him from making more assertive efforts to get new clients.

Therapist and patient realized how much his behavior was inhibited by guilt and self-punishment for angry and competitive feelings, leading them to further explore the developmental origins of these emotions. The earliest and most competitive feelings he recalled were aroused with his older brother. He was angry that his brother was favored, despite his aggressive, bullying behavior. Efforts to compete with his brother were thwarted by his parents, who wanted him to be the "good boy."

> Mr. O: I know that in my efforts at work, I was trying to outdo my brother and show my parents they were wrong about favoring him.
> Therapist: How do you feel about this?
> Mr. O: Well, good at first, but now I feel guilty about it. I mean, I didn't expect things to go so badly for him. I hope I didn't cause any of it.
> Th: How would you have done that?
> Mr. O: I guess by making him feel bad through doing well myself. Maybe I deserve the problems I'm having now.
> Th: As punishment for your outdoing him?
> Mr. O: Yes, in a way.

As he better understood the origin of these conflicts, he began to feel more freedom to be assertive in his office, and made increased efforts to expand his territories. As he felt safer with his competitive wishes, he had a dream in which his rival at work was having difficulty and he felt very happy about it; he acknowledged that he actually enjoyed outdoing others.

Similar to how he felt with his wife and work, Mr. O experienced feelings of inadequacy at times with his therapist, fearing that the clinician wanted him to be more assertive and that he was not getting a "good grade" and was disappointing him. The therapist explored Mr. O's need to be the good patient and submit to what he felt the therapist required of him, just as Mr. O had with his mother: to be the good little boy. Mr. O reported a dream in which his mother asked him whether her hair looked attractive, and he refused to respond to the question. He saw this dream as representing his newfound unwillingness to yield to demands of others. He had felt particularly relieved by being able to discuss the pressures he felt from the therapist. After the exploration of this dream and the therapist's perceived expectations, Mr. O was finally able to confront his wife about their difficulties.

> Mr. O: I asked her whether she believed in monogamy. She was somewhat evasive. I told her that I would be very upset about the idea of her getting involved with another man.
> Th: And how did she respond to that?
> Mr. O: She didn't respond directly at the time, but since then she's been quite solicitous and warmer.
> Th: So confronting her didn't bring the results that you feared.
> Mr. O: No. I guess it was the opposite.

## Working With the Impact of Behavioral Change

Although asserting herself continued to be a struggle at times, Ms. I made progress in addressing her frustration with her husband. Rather than the conflict and hurt she anticipated, her husband increased his efforts to work more consistently and contribute to household chores, and reduced his attempts to restrict her social activities. This helped to diminish her dissatisfaction, anger, and guilt. A similar process occurred at the office, where her increasing critiques of her associates helped reduce her frustration and extra work, while there was little evidence of the pain or humiliation that Ms. I anticipated. These changes eased her overall level of anger and fear, as well as her conflicts about these feelings and fantasies.

Mr. O's wife did not directly deny an affair but became warmer and more responsive, available, and loving. Their sexual relationship improved. He felt more empowered and less inadequate and noted how he had more impact than anticipated. His anger diminished along with the guilt that he felt about his anger, and he stopped expressing it indirectly via going to masseuses or in self-punitive form.

These changes enabled the therapist to address Mr. O's previous perceptions of powerlessness and his shifting views of himself in relation to others.

> Th: You've tended to see your wife as having all the power, while you needed to follow along because of your inadequacies. But it seems different to you now.
> Mr. O: I guess so. I've had more impact on her than I thought I could.
> Th: Rather than being powerless, you actually have a power that you never suspected with her.
> Mr. O: Yes. I really wish I had seen that before. I was so worried that I no longer could have any impact in our relationship.

A shift in Mr. O's representations of himself and others can be noted, from seeing himself as inadequate and his wife as powerful to seeing himself as empowered with a more collaborative relationship with her.

## Making Use of Homework

The concept of homework, a technique commonly used in cognitive-behavioral therapy (Thoma et al. 2015), would be seen as inimical to psychoanalytic treatments, or if employed, would be viewed as part of a supportive psychotherapy. Several principles of psychoanalytic psychotherapy would be seen as adversely affected by homework. The process of tracking thoughts, feelings, and behavior could interfere with free association and access to unconscious content. From this perspective, structuring a session to review homework could collude with patients' resistance to recognizing feelings and conflicts that are painful to them. It could also be viewed as a departure from abstinence and neutrality, with a patient potentially submitting to or rebelling against the homework. However, as with other parameters considered in this book, the actual impact of implementing homework on psychoanalytic psychotherapeutic process is unclear and has not been well studied. The potential value of homework would at least call for a reconsideration of its exclusion from psychodynamic psychotherapeutic approaches.

Indeed, there are several ways in which homework could be of value as a tool in the development of self-exploratory capacities in addition to efforts at behavioral change. For example, one form of homework is keeping a diary, such as that used in certain studies of panic-focused psychodynamic psychotherapy (Busch et al. 2012). Patients note the occurrence of panic attacks, associated symptoms, and the context, feelings, and thoughts associated with the attack. This diary aids in the development of self-monitoring skills in self-exploration, and helps patients to develop the idea that symptoms tend to occur in certain contexts (e.g., separation), with particular feelings and meanings (e.g., angry thoughts and fantasies, separation fears). Therapists can at times review the diaries with patients to identify context, themes, and meanings of symptoms. Recognition of these patterns helps patients gain a sense of control with symptoms that previously felt "out of the blue."

There were no indications in these treatments that the diaries inhibited the process of psychodynamic psychotherapy. Indeed, they may have spurred patients' involvement in treatment as they gained a rapid sense of the value of psychodynamic approaches.

In addition, diaries can help, rather than inhibit, access to patients' painful fears and fantasies by more careful monitoring outside of session. Alertness to their thought process and feelings can tap into meaningful and frightening material that is important to address as it emerges in environments other than the therapeutic setting.

Three core homework approaches are considered for behavioral change in this book. In the first, patients monitor emotions and contexts of particular symptoms and problematic behaviors in diary form. A diary can be used to track thoughts, feelings, and symptoms that arise in the context of attempting to accomplish particular behaviors. This tracking enables patients to bring into therapy what they have identified as they develop their monitoring capacities and attempt to achieve behavioral goals. This information can help identify factors that interfere with accomplishing behavioral change, such as particular feelings, conflicts, defenses, and fantasies. Furthermore, it can aid in the discussion of strategies to counter interfering factors at the point of attempting the behavior.

In a second type of homework the therapist works with the patient in developing a written psychodynamic formulation that can be updated over the course of the therapy. This process can help the patient to keep in mind a growing understanding of how his mind works and affects his feelings and behaviors. Third, patients can make a written note of certain potential scripts, what they anticipate the response of others will be, what interferes with enacting these scripts, and what their response and that of others is to actual use of the script. Thus the patient can keep in mind and report to the therapist the impact and experience of their efforts at particular behavioral interventions.

## Case Example

Ms. P, a 32-year-old editor, struggled with setting limits with her father, who was recurrently bullying and abusive to her, despite her becoming more empowered and improving in many areas of her life. Several factors contributed, including a recurrent hope that somehow he would change his behavior and not behave abusively. However, he consistently would attack the patient unfairly, such as stating that she did not pay enough attention to him and his girlfriend. Sometimes the attacks were more general and the content was unclear; he simply acted irritated with her. The patient continued to feel badly about being bullied by him and wanted to find some way to heal their relationship. However, after their visits she would end up deeply disappointed and depressed. She considered ending the visits but feared he might cut off contact with her.

> Therapist: So it's very difficult for you to avoid getting together with him.
> 
> Ms. P: Yes, I know. I keep hoping for change in spite of his behavior. I'm not sure what to do. I really want to stop this pattern.
> 
> Th: I think you should consider taking the stance that you won't spend time with him unless he treats you differently. So you don't keep exposing yourself to his bullying.
> 
> Ms. P: How could I do that?
> 
> Th: I think we should have you write a note that he has to stop criticizing you or losing his temper. That you'll end the visit or conversation if he doesn't behave differently.
> 
> Ms. P: Well, that does sound empowering. How do we know I'll be able to stick with that plan?
> 
> Th: We have to see if you feel safe with it and try to understand what the conflict is if you don't. This will put some structure in your decisions to get together and allow us a better opportunity to explore them.
> 
> Ms. P: I'd be very interested in doing that. But what if he reacts badly to it?
> 
> Th: Of course that's possible, but accepting the current situation is not helping you. I think the best thing would be for you

to write up what you might say or present to your father. And let's see how you feel about it.

Ms. P: Yes, I'd like to try that. I think I would feel better about myself if I do it that way.

Writing this note not only helped Ms. P overcome her inhibitions and clarify limits, but also was effective in modifying her father's behavior. She sent it as a letter to her father, which described specific behaviors that were unacceptable and indicated that the patient would leave the house and not recontact him if he breached the rules. Surprisingly to her, her father took the letter seriously and agreed to abide by it. Indeed, Ms. P would refer to the note when her father began to act again in a problematic way, such as when he became critical of her, which would stop the behavior from escalating.

Extensive tweaking of behavioral shifts is often required as patients steadily confront inhibitory fears and assess the impact on others. Although in most instances others are ultimately supportive and responsive, in some instances they may persistently ignore or show antagonism toward patients' efforts. The maintenance of such problematic relationships needs to be explored, as it can indicate a fear of loss of attachment, a recurrently disappointed fantasy that the relationship can somehow be "fixed," and/or the persistence of guilt. Indeed, sometimes a patient's health is best aided when he or she reduces contact or withdraws from a relationship that is inherently damaging. These problematic responses will be explored in greater depth in Chapter 9 ("Working With Sustaining Behavioral Change and the Response of Others").

# References

Busch FN, Milrod BL, Singer M, et al: Panic-Focused Psychodynamic Psychotherapy—eXtended Range. New York, Routledge, 2012

Busch FN, Rudden MG, Shapiro T: Psychodynamic Treatment of Depression, 2nd Edition. Arlington, VA, American Psychiatric Publishing, 2016

Thoma N, Pilecki B, McKay D: Contemporary cognitive behavior therapy: a review of theory, history, and evidence. Psychodyn Psychiatry 43(3):423–461, 2015 26301761

# 6

# Identifying Dynamic Contributors to Problematic Behaviors

In targeting behavioral change, the therapist works with the patient to articulate the context, feelings, and thoughts that precede problematic actions and inhibitions (Table 6–1). To better examine these elements, the therapist aids the patient in developing self-observational capacities. Using the information about situational and emotional triggers, the therapist helps to identify dynamic contributors to the avoidance or enactment of certain behaviors, including uncomfortable or frightening fantasies, intrapsychic conflicts, defense mechanisms, and relevant developmental and traumatic events. These approaches enable the development of a psychodynamic formulation or framework that aids in devising strategies for changing behavior. In many instances several factors need to be addressed for the patient to gain greater control over problematic behavior.

## Development of Self-Observational Capacity

The process of examining factors surrounding behavioral problems benefits from the development of self-observational capacity, which, as noted in Chapter 2 ("Understanding Psychodynamic Factors That Impede Behavioral Change"), is considered an aspect of mentalization (Busch

**TABLE 6–1.** Examining the context, affects, and meanings of problematic behavior

Developing the capacity for self-observation
    Psychoeducation about this skill
    Metaphors: scaffolding/reviewing a videotape
    Use of this technique in therapy
    Recognition of disruptions to this capacity: conflicts, painful feelings, trauma
Identifying the circumstances in which the behavior occurs
Considering relevant developmental and/or traumatic events
Exploring the affects and fantasies that precede the inhibition or behavior
Establishing the meanings and psychodynamics surrounding the inhibition or behavior
Identifying multiple contributors to behavior

2008). This monitoring of mental states is often a skill that patients need to be taught or learn to use more frequently. This ability is enhanced through the therapist's approach, in which identification of internal experiences and environmental circumstances is repeatedly emphasized. In addition, use of a diary to monitor context, thought, feelings, and behavior, as discussed in Chapter 5 ("Establishing a Framework for Targeting Behavioral Change"), can be of value.

Metaphors can be useful ways to communicate about the process of self-observation and for examining triggers relevant to behavioral change. One way of describing the monitoring of personal intrapsychic states and behavioral patterns is with the notion of "building a scaffold." With a scaffold in place patients can examine their feelings and behavior more closely to identify problems and their sources, just as a scaffold allows closer and safer observation and access to a structure that needs to be modified. The development of self-observational capacities and a psychodynamic formulation aids in the process of change or repair of aspects of the self and behavior. Another way of describing this stance is to discuss reviewing a videotape surrounding certain behaviors to see how one is feeling and reacting to the relevant circumstances. New strategies can be derived and tested based on this analysis. Both metaphors emphasize the concept of stepping back and evaluating with an observing ego.

Therapists and patients should also be on the alert for factors that can disrupt the capacity for self-observation. These elements can include shame, anxiety, conflicts, or trauma linked to what the patient is addressing at that time. Disruptions in self-observation can also function as a defensive form of "not knowing" to avoid painful or frightening thoughts and fantasies. Therapists can call attention to a sudden interruption in self-observation as an indicator of emotions or conflicts that should be explored.

The following vignette provides an example of examining feelings and thoughts preceding Mr. E's (the accountant discussed in Chapter 3, "Identifying and Addressing Risks in Targeting Behavioral Change") tendency to become distracted and procrastinate when he is attempting to focus on his work. The therapist noted the presence of a specific disruption in self-observational capacity.

> Mr. E: I know I'm supposed to be focused on finding new clients, but then I just get distracted by other things. I think I'll just spend a few minutes on them and I end up spending an hour or two.
> Therapist: Can you tell me more about what happens? It would be good to get some specific examples to look at.
> Mr. E: I'm such an idiot. I should be working consistently, and I get caught up in these things.

This self-criticism provides an example of a specific type of interference with self-examination of behaviors. Patients can experience such a powerful sense of shame, anxiety, or guilt surrounding certain actions that their capacity to think about them is unconsciously derailed, inadvertently contributing to the persistence of the behavior. Mr. E's harsh self-view immediately blocks him from being able to step back and consider causal factors. The therapist can identify this pattern and explore the nature of the patient's negative feelings. In recent sessions, they had been exploring developmental experiences surrounding his father's harsh judgments and criticisms of himself and others, which proved relevant to his current reaction.

> Th: Why do you think you're so self-critical about getting distracted?
> Mr. E: I'm not sure. I'm embarrassed. I should have more control.
> Th: Well, it seems like a big overreaction in terms of self-criticism. Procrastination is a common problem, and we're trying to understand

more about how it operates with you. Maybe the intense criticism comes from something else.

Mr. E: Well, as I said, my father was very critical. Maybe that has something to do with it?

Th: It probably does. We'll need to help you understand more about how his attitudes could lead to attacks on yourself and how it then interferes with your focus on tasks.

## Identifying Developmental and Traumatic Events as Contributors to Problematic Behaviors

Painful developmental events and trauma are often found to be sources of behavioral problems. Examining the context of behaviors can often be used to identify relevant past links to these experiences. For example, Mr. E's experience of feeling criticized and rejected by his father related to the threat he felt when contacting colleagues. The relevance of adverse and traumatic events, discussed in greater depth in Chapter 11 ("Addressing Behavioral Problems Related to Adverse Developmental Experiences and Trauma"), may be difficult to identify because of repression or dissociation of these painful experiences, but can be strongly linked to behavioral inhibitions as well as impulsive behaviors. Identifying these events and how they relate to the patient's feelings, conflicts, and actions is of significant value in targeting behavioral change, as discussed in the case examples in the following section involving procrastination and angry behavior.

## Identifying the Circumstances, Feelings, and Meanings Surrounding Problematic Behavior: Procrastination

The elaboration of the context, affects, and meanings of behavior allows for the development of a framework for understanding and intervention, as in the case of Mr. E's procrastination. These situations and emotional states typically act as triggers for the behavior, and recognizing them helps to identify contributing fantasies, conflicts, and developmental factors that can be addressed by the therapist. In the case of Mr. E, the therapist had obtained a history about developmental events that remained deeply upsetting to Mr. E. A contentious divorce when the patient was age 11 led to him and his two brothers moving with his mother to a smaller house and a different school, and he recalled that after the move his father made little effort to maintain a relationship with him. The therapist was able to identify the relevance of these experiences to his current struggles with procrastination.

> Th: I think it's important to consider and discuss what you experience at the point when you get distracted. First, we can look at what goes on inside that triggers moving away from your work. Then we can start to build a scaffold from which to consider what happens and identify ways to prevent it. Do you have a specific example?
>
> Mr. E: Okay. Well, I was about to call a colleague I needed to talk to in order to get some advice, and then I got distracted about my doctor not calling me back after I called him. I started to write an e-mail complaining to the doctor and it got longer and longer. I didn't end up making the call. I was so angry with myself about it.
>
> Th: That seems to fit in with some issues we've talked about. You become preoccupied with situations in which others are not being responsive to your needs, and you feel a sense of injustice.
>
> Mr. E: Yeah. Definitely. I don't get how a doctor can just not call you back. What if something is really wrong?
>
> Th: Well, that's a good point. And what comes to mind about the call you were going to make about help finding additional work?
>
> Mr. E: Well, I'm not sure if the guy I'm reaching out to is really going to be helpful to me. In fact, he might be dismissive or even ask why I'm bothering him. I guess it does remind me of what we talked about regarding my father the other day, about being afraid of him. And I just felt like a burden, like I was keeping him from doing what he wanted.
>
> Th: These reactions do sound like your experience of your father when you were an adolescent. You had described fears of his criticizing you, but not that you were burdensome. I wonder if that was part of your feelings?
>
> Mr. E: Well, I guess so. He did seem like he was involved in his new life. He was busy with work and dating, and not too shortly after he met the woman who became my stepmom. But you know, I really should just be able make these calls.
>
> Th: That's why we're trying to understand more: being self-critical or knowing you should do it hasn't really helped that much. Painful feelings surge up when you're about to call, and you deal with them in part by pushing them out of your mind and procrastinating.
>
> Mr. E: Yeah, well, I recognize now I get embarrassed and anxious about asking a colleague for help. I think they'll just blow me off.

> Th: But your colleagues have generally been very receptive. The response you expect sounds more like your experience with your father. Maybe that's why you think they'll react so negatively. You might want to consider that your expectations are overly negative at that point.
>
> Mr. E: Okay, I'll try to do that.

Ms. B (Chapter 2) procrastinated as she struggled to start writing papers for graduate school, reporting anxiety and pressure, leading her to do other chores. When asked what came to mind when she experienced this tension, she recalled the period in which her father put increasing pressure on her and her brother to perform at school. He got furious when the brother received a B on an important test and ranted about how they would not get into an Ivy League college if they did not study harder. His rages about academic performance came at a time when he had switched from working at a financial firm to being a real estate agent. However, he was struggling to make sales, and the family began to be affected financially. Ms. B stated that he increasingly wanted to "live through us" with regard to his pressuring them to achieve. She shifted from enjoying her schoolwork to feeling anxious and preoccupied. The therapist suggested that when she started to write Ms. B appeared to be in the state of mind she had during this difficult time period in her past.

> Th: It seems like before you sit down to write that you're feeling the way you felt at that time in your life. You feel pressured and worried that you're not smart enough and that it will be catastrophic if you can't write well. After you start it seems like you're at the point in your life where you enjoyed writing.
>
> Ms. B: It's interesting because as you say that it feels like the pressure I'm experiencing is the same I had at that time. My father was obsessed with us doing well in school and it was just so uncomfortable. It seemed like he would go crazy if we didn't get an A.
>
> Th: So it's consistent with the patterns we've talked about in other situations. You have to give up your needs or even your own enjoyment to respond to your parents' or others' wishes and feelings. In this case you had to manage your father's sense of inadequacy and diminishing self-esteem by doing well. You believed it was necessary to rescue him, just as you had to respond to your mother's pressures about your appearance.
>
> Ms. B: Yes, I guess I just get stuck in that place. But I'm not sure how to get out once I'm stuck there.

Th: One option is setting a time to start. Then we'll have more information about what you're experiencing when that time is approaching. Then we can address the feelings and thoughts that are directly inhibiting you. Another option is touching base with your mentor at the time you start writing. This helps you feel connected with someone who is supportive, who encourages your writing.

Ms. B: Okay, I'll try to set a time and see when my mentor might be available to touch base.

One factor guiding the therapist's recommendation about Ms. B's procrastination relates to the value of connecting with another supportive person. Many patients struggle with feelings of aloneness when taking on a task and feel unable to get any help from others. In addition, they believe that if they seek support, others will not be responsive to their needs or will be critical or rejecting, often based on developmental experiences. Employing this formulation as developed with Ms. B, the therapist believed she could overcome her inhibition by engaging someone who responded positively to her efforts. This relationship could provide "evidence" that she was not in the same circumstances she was previously. Indeed, Ms. B was able to rapidly get involved with her writing when working with her mentor.

## Identifying the Context, Fantasies, and Emotions Triggering Angry Behavior

Many individuals and patients complain of difficulties with control of angry feelings and behaviors. Some patients are overinhibited about expressing angry feelings or lack access to them, whereas others have difficulty limiting the intensity of their expressions of anger, as with temper outbursts. Alternatively, patients can be overly inhibited in certain circumstances and lack impulse control in others. The effort to identify circumstances, feelings, and meanings surrounding anger can aid patients in expressing it in a more effective manner. Clarifying triggers can also help build a mental space for patients to pause and consider before acting.

Ms. F, the 48-year-old nurse discussed in Chapter 3, had struggled for many years with her son's demands, which would cause feelings of anxiety and guilt, and a pressure to respond to his expressions of need. Over the course of her therapeutic work she became more aware of her anger at him in these circumstances. However, at first it emerged in such an intense form that she reported not being able to think. She shifted between an inability to say anything to her son to comments that were more severe and hurtful than she intended, such as "You're a terrible kid." The therapist and patient explored the triggers of her feelings, which included her son's harsh criticisms of her and aggressive refusals to do something she asked. They considered her own history, and in particular how she felt obligated to respond to her parents' needs while eschewing her own and felt any expression of anger toward them was ineffective and pointless. The therapist worked with Ms. F to help her identify what she was experiencing in her mind when she felt angry, with a goal of managing it more effectively. The therapist had used the concept of reviewing a videotape to encourage Ms. F to examine what was occurring when her rage was triggered.

> Ms. F: I paid attention to what was making me angry and I'm reviewing it like a tape as you suggested. I became aware it's really his lack of empathy and unwillingness to accept any responsibility when we're fighting. He'll say, "I need a ride," and if I try to say no because I'm meeting a friend, he'll say, "What am I supposed to do then? Don't you even care about my having a social life?"
> Th: I certainly understand your frustration at that point. What do you think stops you from saying something to him?
> Ms. F: If I say anything, he just attacks that. He doesn't take any responsibility or own up to his role in a fight. So if I say I can't do it because I'm meeting a friend, he'll say, "So it's all about you."
> Th: I think your ability to define what infuriates you better gives us some clues as to how to better manage the conflict with him. You might want to say, when he's calmer, that when you can't give him what he wants he gets angry very fast and has trouble considering your perspective.
> Ms. F: Okay, well I'm not sure that's going to work even when he's calmer. And it might just get him mad again.
> Th: Well, that may be, but I think you are also used to the tensions you felt with your parents. They made very unfair attacks on you and were also not open to discussing things, so I think you assume that Sam will always be the same.
> Ms. F: Well, also he's been this way a long time. I just expect a fight.
> Th: I'm sure that contributes.

Using the metaphor of reviewing a videotape, Ms. F's capacity to observe what triggered her rage and what she experienced when she was angry led to a more defined understanding of what her son said that made her furious, why it made her angry, and what developmental factors had contributed to her reaction. This understanding provided a framework that had been absent when her rage emerged when struggling with him. The therapist also suggested that she talk with her son when they were not involved in an altercation. In many instances in which problematic behavior emerges, there is an avoidance of a discussion between episodes of conflict. Part of this avoidance may be based on concerns about "rocking the boat" by raising an area of potential conflict when tensions are at an ebb. These concerns should be explored, as addressing problems when tensions are diminished is often a valuable intervention for behavioral change.

## Identifying Dynamic Factors Contributing to Problematic Behavior

Using the information about context and emotions, the therapist helps the patient to identify dynamic contributors to problematic behaviors, working to further develop a framework for understanding and intervention. These factors include uncomfortable or frightening fantasies, intrapsychic conflicts, and defense mechanisms. In the case of Mr. E, for example, the therapist and patient discussed the relevance of his father's criticisms and disregard of him when he was young to his negative expectations from colleagues. In addition, procrastination functioned in part as a defense against painful anxieties about being judged as inadequate. The vignette below provides additional historical information aiding in the development of a psychodynamic formulation.

> In the course of treatment, Mr. E had become more alert to when he felt the urge to put off a call to help him find new business, allowing him to identify better what he was experiencing:
>
> > Mr. E: I'm aware now of this other resistance to calling. I just don't feel I should have to do it. I feel like I should just be taken care of by others.
> > Th: How do you understand this?
> > Mr. E: I think it's not really fair that I should have to put out all this effort when it's so stressful for me to build my business. Others just seem to get taken care of. They don't have any financial problems or they just have connections that get them work.
> > Th: You mean the insiders and outsiders? You feel some people have these connections and wealth.

Mr. E: Yes. And I recognize that I actually have a lot. I mean I have family members that can help. And my wife works. But it still feels this way. And I'm mad about it.

Th: I think it's so important to be aware of the wish to be taken care of and your sense of unfairness, as those feelings contribute to a wish to rebel against your work efforts. I think procrastinating is a way of expressing your anger indirectly. And I believe it interferes under the radar. You're often not aware of when it takes effect. If we understand more about it you could limit its impact. It seems like your feelings are reminiscent of what happened when your father got divorced and you had to move with your mother.

Mr. E: Well, that's true. It was when I was 11, which I guess was a vulnerable time. But I definitely went from a place where we had a fancy lifestyle to one where it was very different. My mom made it clear that we had to watch every penny. I guess there were fights with my dad about child support. And my dad wasn't very involved with me. He paid more attention to my brother, who was an athlete.

Th: So the sense of unfairness comes partly from thinking about what you had before and feeling jealous of others who have more.

Mr. E: Yes, and what my father still had. I mean, I didn't think about it that way then. I imagined how my friends, whom I missed, were enjoying some of the things I used to do. And I didn't like the new school I went to either. I didn't know any kids and I really didn't fit in there. I was very upset.

Th: Well, one thing that's clear is that you're still upset about it. And it's part of what leads you to believe that you're not going to get additional work because you're not connected. Or somehow it should just be given to you!

Mr. E: Definitely. It's not very realistic.

Th: So it's important to keep an eye out for these feelings and ideas interfering with your job-seeking efforts, as not having more work causes you to feel even more frustrated and deprived.

Mr. E: That's true. Well I did push through it and set up a meeting.

Th: That's a very encouraging example of using this information.

In this instance the therapist offered the patient a preliminary formulation, suggesting that Mr. E's expectation of being disregarded and criticized stemmed from his early history. Mr. E's experiences and associated perceptions contributed to his feelings of inadequacy and also his anger at others for putting pressure on him to work. He procrastinated to avoid feeling embarrassed or attacked, a form of defense, and this behavior indirectly expressed his anger at those he believed were responsible for this pressure. Pursuing distractions, however, ultimately exacerbated his feelings of inadequacy and anger, as it interfered with his capacity to build his business. By helping to recognize and tolerate his feelings of inadequacy and anger, as well as their origins, this framework could be employed to help the patient avert his tendency to procrastinate.

As discussed earlier in this chapter, Ms. F struggled with her own feelings toward her parents, contributing to the development of tensions with her son. Ms. F felt pressure to submit to her parents' needs, expecting to be harshly criticized or abandoned if she did not do so. She suppressed her anger at them, believing any expression of it could lead to being rejected or triggering their fury. In part she put her son in the position of her parents, believing she must submit to his needs or be attacked. If she experienced angry feelings and attempted to set limits with him, she viewed herself as being harsh and damaging as her parents were to her, a form of identification with the aggressor. This framework helped to untangle the factors that led to her problematic struggle with anger.

> Ms. F: I think another reason that I'm frightened of my anger toward him is that I worry he's too vulnerable.
> Th: What do you think would happen?
> Ms. F: I'm not really sure. If he doesn't get his way he gets so upset!
> Th: Well, I really wonder if he would get as upset as you expect if you stuck with a limit. Also, I'm not sure what damage you anticipate. When there are limits on his behavior at school he seems to be able to deal with them.
> Ms. F: That's true. Although occasionally he's argued with teachers.
> Th: But he's never been punished for that. I think there is a pattern in part of you seeing him like your parents, and you fear retaliation from him when you get angry. However, another part of you fears damaging him if you get mad or set limits. It's important to understand these different struggles you have, as you end up feeling anxious and confused.
> Ms. F: Well I think I understand what you're saying. I want to understand more about these different parts of myself. I think I would be less frightened and could sort this out better.

## Developing the Framework Further by Examining Multiple Contributors

Part of the persistence of problematic behavior stems from the existence of multiple contributors and functions, as in the cases above. Clinicians should recognize that they will likely identify additional factors after an initial psychodynamic formulation, and should be particularly alert if there is a lack of change after determining a behavioral trigger and suggesting alternative actions. An ongoing examination of the context, emotions, and meanings surrounding behavioral problems aids in further development of the formulation of fantasies, conflicts, and developmental factors. This effort, part of the working through process (see Chapter 4, "Using Psychodynamic Techniques in Addressing Behavioral Change" for description), helps develop additional points of intervention to avert problematic behaviors.

> ### Case Example
> 
> Ms. Q, a 69-year-old female therapist, described frustration with her children's lack of responsiveness to her efforts to seek support from them about her wish for more help now that she was aging. It emerged over time, however, that she was actually not revealing to them what her needs were, such as assistance with certain tasks. Her fears of expressing her anger, which had inhibited her from addressing her concerns and frustrations with them, had been identified (see Chapter 7, "Identifying Alternative Behaviors"). Although she was now more comfortable expressing angry feelings, this had not helped to change her behavior. On further exploration of the context and feelings, the therapist and Ms. Q were able to determine that she was conflicted about revealing her needs to them, in part related to conflicts about seeking support and her developmental experiences.
> 
> > Ms. Q: I'm still frustrated that my kids don't recognize that I'm getting older and that I need more help. They don't ask how I'm doing or if I need anything.
> > Th: I know we've discussed that before and recognized that you feared getting too angry with them. You were going to set up a meeting with them to discuss your needs and your feelings. What happened when you tried to do that?
> > Ms. Q: Well, that's true that I was planning to set up a meeting. It's almost like I forgot. Thinking about it, I realize it's difficult for me to bring it up because I feel vulnerable talking

*Identifying Dynamic Contributors to Problematic Behaviors*             85

> about getting older. I've always been independent. I've made it clear I didn't need help.
>
> Th: Why do you think you've been like this?
>
> Ms. Q: I always had to take care of my mother. She was always panicking about her health, always catastrophic. It was almost like I was the mother and she was the kid. I think I grew up kind of fast. And I didn't want to do this to my kids!
>
> Th: But now you do want more support, but you're in conflict about it. You seem to be equating any asking for help to behaving like your mother. You really haven't told them you need help and they're not used to responding to you in this way. We have to understand more about your fears of being vulnerable, and you're going to have to develop a language to communicate to them about what help you need.
>
> Ms. Q: I'm not really sure how to do this.
>
> Th: So, I actually do think you have an idea of how to approach this. You've told me previously you were going to discuss your medical problems and what help you might need from them. I think it would be good to set up the meeting and be on the alert for urges you have to cancel it.
>
> Ms. Q: I think I'm worried about losing my independence. I have a friend whose daughter does everything for her. But she really likes it.
>
> Th: I think this is one of the problems. You tend to think about this as all or none. Either you're completely helpless, like your mother or friend, and lose all independence, or completely independent, not getting any help at all.
>
> Ms. Q: I see that I get scared and make the situation black or white. Then I avoid it. I'll talk to them again about scheduling the meeting. If I find myself avoiding it again I'll see what else comes up and we can talk more about it.

A growing formulation and framework provided a more complex understanding and a broader range of interventions for the patient's difficulty engaging her children. This example also demonstrates the value of identifying an alternative behavioral goal, such as a meeting with the children, as discussed in the next chapter. If the patient is intent on changing a behavior but does not do so, the therapist can explore what inhibited them from taking the alternative step, in this instance fears of being vulnerable and losing her independence.

## Reference

Busch FN (ed): Mentalization: Theoretical Considerations, Research Findings, and Clinical Implications. Hillsdale, NJ, Analytic Press, 2008

# Identifying Alternative Behaviors

In a significant departure from traditional psychodynamic psychotherapy, the therapist targeting behavioral change works with patients to identify alternative behaviors. These approaches include discussing the employment of specific actions, or "scripts," in addressing problems with others. In addition to behavioral difficulties caused by intrapsychic conflicts and other dynamic factors, patients may have had limited exposure to effective strategies for managing problems in close attachment relationships. Oftentimes they grew up in circumstances in which anger and needs were poorly managed, with frequent blaming or shaming of family members. Suggesting potential interventions can help build a repertoire of strategies to ease interpersonal conflicts and for patients to recognize that it is possible to do so. The therapeutic relationship also provides a model of how to talk about strong feelings and problems without being judged or criticized.

As with other interventions suggested in this book, considering alternative behaviors can aid, rather than disrupt, a psychoanalytic treatment. An understanding of the dynamics that contribute to problematic behaviors can help identify strategies for change, and discussing possible alternatives can provide new insights. Considering new options allows

**TABLE 7–1.** Identifying alternative behaviors

Using the collaborative approach
Behavioral examples
    Setting limits
    Directly addressing problems with others
Using scripts

for more direct exploration of factors that interfere with making behavioral changes (see Chapter 8, "Identifying Interfering Factors in Performing Alternative Behaviors"). There are no set rules for identifying alternatives, and therapists typically work with patients to make these determinations. This chapter will describe examples of considering behavioral strategies and the use of scripts.

# Using the Collaborative Approach

## Setting Limits

Limit setting, discussed further in Chapter 10 ("Engaging the Patient in Specific Behavioral Problems"), is a common area of behavioral difficulties. Oftentimes patients are not aware of how to set limits with others in a way that is not excessively timid or overly harsh. Problems managing anger and anxiety often emerge as contributors to these difficulties, as patients worry about being hostile or triggering the ire of the other person. Patients benefit from suggestions about strategies to establish boundaries that are firm but not overly severe. In the case example below, Ms. R struggled with managing angry feelings and comments alternating with an overly permissive stance toward her children, but she was not consciously aware of these shifts and changes. The therapist suggested a series of clear limits with potential consequences if not followed, but discussed presenting them in a way that was not overly attacking.

### Case Example

Ms. R, a divorced 48-year-old paralegal, struggled with frustrations with her college-age children, a boy and girl, believing them to be lazy and uncaring. She thought neither would find jobs and that they would live "forever" in the family home, all the while maintaining a sullen attitude toward her. She was frustrated by their lack of participation in regular household chores and abrogation of her rules regarding cleanliness or curfews. She alternated between threats of cutting off any funds or kicking them out of the house and an overly tolerant, accepting attitude. Ms. R was unaware how her own anger might contribute to her children's attitude toward her and responsibilities.

> Therapist: I think you might not recognize that when you don't address a problem for a while they may think it's okay to do it. And then you get furious when you become aware of it again and your stance becomes very harsh. It's certainly one thing to address problems in their behavior, but it's another to threaten to stop paying for food and kick them out. I think you may not be aware of how angry you feel, and the way you express it exacerbates the tensions between you and them.
> Ms. R: Yes. I feel like they just don't care about me at all. And I feel helpless. If I don't threaten to throw them out, what would work? I'll just be stuck with them.
> Th: Well, I think we need to understand more about why you feel it's hopeless with them. They struggle with getting schoolwork or job searches done and about rules, but we need to understand more about why you believe it's hopeless. There are several ways of handling it that we can discuss. One would be to identify a series of steps that they would need to take, with more specific consequences if they don't follow them. Another would be to try more positive approaches, such as meeting them for lunch and discussing their plans.
> Ms. R: I'm happy to talk about those options, but I'm not sure they'll be effective.

Ms. R described a background in which she was viewed as the most rebellious of the family. Her parents, who divorced when she was 8, were very involved in their own activities: her father with business and her mother with social events. Ms. R believed she would break rules primarily to get her parents' attention, which she could not otherwise obtain. However, even this defiance brought only a very brief focus on her, with minimal consequences, and a subsequent return to feeling disregarded. Over time she recognized that she struggled with a feeling of hopeless anger toward her parents.

> Th: Well, I wonder to some extent if it reminds you of your own frustrated rebellion and attention seeking, and your children may feel reminiscent of your parents, unresponsive

>   to your concerns. You end up feeling stuck, but your manner of expressing your feelings only creates more distance.
>
> Ms. R: That sounds right. I'd like to talk more about that.
>
> Th: I agree we should. And in the meantime the suggestions I'm making offer you more opportunities of communicating and responding to them, which you felt was lacking so much in your adolescence and college years.
>
> Ms. R: Okay. I've been trying to use these strategies a bit more. They were interested in going out to dinner to talk about things. I was surprised.

Further information can be obtained about a patient by assessing how others respond to behavioral options. When the therapist initially suggested to Ms. R that she have a positive discussion with her son about his plans, her frustration became more apparent.

> Ms. R: I don't think it's going to help. I don't think he's going to get a job. He never worked before college.
>
> Th: Why would that mean he would not get a job now?
>
> Ms. R: He just hasn't shown any interest. And if he stays home he won't pay rent. There won't be any way to pressure him to work. I'll have to force him to leave
>
> Th: Well, at a certain point you can let him know that if he's going to live with you he'll need to get a job.
>
> Ms. R: I think he'll just refuse. And then I'm not sure what I'd do.
>
> Th: I think that this is a catastrophic scenario. I'm not saying it couldn't happen. But he could get a job after he finishes school or he could get one when you made it clear that he needed to if he wanted to live in the house. You're already believing you will get in a struggle about him moving out. I think we need to understand more about why you would see him this way. Who might he represent for you? Perhaps your parents when they were focused on their own activities and were unresponsive or critical of you?
>
> Ms. R: I'm not sure. It doesn't feel too negative to me. It feels accurate. But I hear what you're saying. In a sense my parents ignored their responsibilities toward me, just as I feel the kids are.

An example of discussing behavioral options and developing psychodynamic understanding emerged in her recognition of hopelessness, causing her to dismiss potential options and to anticipate a negative outcome of her efforts. Determining the roots of her sense of hopelessness in her childhood experience helped her to recognize a greater potential to change the circumstances with her own children.

## Directly Addressing Problems

Many patients struggle with directly addressing their concerns with others. They may fear they will attack others, that others will be rejecting and the relationship will be disrupted, or that they will receive an inadequate response. The therapist can initially encourage patients to address their concerns with new behaviors and then assess inhibitions about doing so. Ultimately, if patients continue to struggle with trying new options to manage a persistent problem, they may benefit from a discussion of scripts (see below). As in other areas of behavioral suggestions, the therapist acknowledges that directly addressing problems is a sensitive task, and the therapist and patient cannot be certain of the best approach and how the other person will react. However, leaving the situation as is can be emotionally untenable for the patient or destructive over the long term. In the example below, the therapist encourages the patient to discuss problems at work with his boss, with the aid of dynamic information.

### Case Example

Mr. S was a 43-year-old businessman being treated in psychotherapy and with escitalopram for anxiety and depression. He had been very worried about a new situation at his job, in which he worked separately from the rest of his group in another city. He was anxious and frustrated about not getting adequate feedback or support from them. He found his therapy of limited value until he had a "revelation" about the degree to which he felt neglected by his parents and how greatly that led him to accept mistreatment or disregard from others. He presented at the session described below complaining of tiredness and motivational problems.

> Mr. S: Work had been going better, but lately I've been stuck sorting out an assignment. I could really use help from others, but I've had a lot of trouble getting it. It's very frustrating.
> Th: How long has that been going on?
> Mr. S: A couple of weeks.
> Th: So I wonder how much the tiredness might be related to that frustration.
> Mr. S: Well, that's possible. It's been very difficult.
> Th: Have you tried to address the problem with your boss?
> Mr. S: Somewhat, but I don't get much of a response.

Th: I wonder how much it might be connected to your feelings of neglect growing up. I'm wondering whether you should step up your efforts to get others to respond to the problem. You could simply tell him that you're not getting the support you need and he can help you with that.
Mr. S: Maybe I should talk more to my boss.
Th: Have you found that difficult to do?
Mr. S: Old habits die hard. Growing up I learned to just try to deal with the problem myself.
Th: Do you feel that if you talked to your boss you wouldn't get a response anyway?
Mr. S: Definitely.
Th: Your tiredness seems to represent something about your being stuck back with your parents, unable to get support. Maybe even the effort of speaking to your boss will help you to feel better.
Mr. S: Okay. Well, that makes sense. I'll try talking to him.

Another component that emerged in Mr. S's therapy was that tiredness and low motivation defended against rageful feelings and fantasies toward his parents and others who were neglectful. An understanding of this rage, along with a growing sense of how to manage it better, helped him feel safer addressing feelings of neglect with others.

## Using Scripts

As noted earlier in this chapter, in this type of dynamically focused behavioral treatment, it can sometimes be valuable to provide patients with "scripts" that contain specific suggestions of what the patient might say or how they might act in a given situation. Oftentimes a script is useful because patients have difficulties identifying or maintaining awareness of comments that might be effective at modulating interpersonal difficulties, either based on their history or because of intrapsychic conflict and anxiety. These scripts are derived from the patients' personal circumstances and dynamics as well as the therapist's own experience in dealing with relationships. The therapist and patients should discuss that the outcome of the use of these scripts is uncertain, and that patients should feel comfortable not using a script the therapist suggests. The development of alternatives is a collaborative effort in which the patient is encouraged to consider other modes of expressing similar comments or ideas.

The patient's reaction to considering the use of a script is of value and can aid in identifying her dynamics and conflicts. The discussion of a specific script can trigger anxiety, as the statements typically express what the patient is fearful of, such as an assertive comment. Sometimes it is useful for the therapist or patient to write down a particular suggestion as the patient may have difficulty remembering it after the session, often because of intrapsychic conflict. Struggles with or avoidance of using the scripted material, even when patients have good intentions, is a further opportunity to explore fears.

## Case Example

Ms. F (see Chapters 3 and 6) frequently struggled with setting limits with her son, and would be upended by his aggressive comments.

> Ms. F: I keep getting furious with him. At first it's a reasonable debate about what he wants. But then he starts screaming and saying, "You don't love me. You don't care about me." Then I get really flustered.
> Th: I think you've been through this plenty of times. I know you still struggle with feeling blamed and guilty. But I think by this point it's worth mentioning something about his saying how you don't love him and care about him. You can reassure him that it's not true and you're sorry if he feels that way. But you're not going to change your mind about a limit based on his saying this.
> Ms. F: That sounds like a good idea, but it may be hard for me. I'm so easily provoked.
> Th: That's why I think it would be helpful for you and him to discuss this ahead of time, when you're not in the midst of a fight. Also you could try writing it down, as it's hard for you to remember in the midst of an argument.
> Ms. F: Yes, I think I will write down that comment you're suggesting. I get so frustrated I can't think of what to say.

## Case Example

Ms. Q (see Chapter 6) struggled with how to express her frustration toward her daughter about what she experienced as neglect, lack of interest, or an unwillingness to help her now that she was getting older. The patient acknowledged that she had difficulty communicating when she needed help from her daughter and that this might be contributing to the problem. However, she wrestled with her anger toward her daughter, which likely contributed to her struggles to directly confront her. Additionally, the way that she planned to address the problem would usually be in a very angry manner, and the therapist and patient were concerned that this would risk alienating her daughter.

Ms. Q: I'm just so frustrated with her. I feel she doesn't care about me. She just ignores me. And she has no interest in my health. I think I have to talk to her about it.

Th: I certainly understand your frustration, although we've talked about how you might both contribute to the problem, and that your daughter does spend time with you. But what would you say?

Ms. Q: I would say, "I think that you don't want to get together and you don't have a kind word for me and I want to understand why."

Th: Well, I'm concerned that your daughter might hear that as an accusation and feel judged. It could get her back up.

Ms. Q: You're probably right. What would you suggest?

Th: Something like, "I feel you don't want to get together with me. I wonder if something's bothering you," or, "I'd like to talk to you more about my health problems but it's difficult for me, and I'm worried you won't want to talk about them."

Ms. Q: Well, those are a lot better. Can you write them down for me?

Th: Sure. But I think you have difficulty controlling and managing your anger and that you see her somewhat like your mother: you have to take care of her needs and not express your concerns. Then you get angry because it feels like she's disregarding you, like your mother.

Ms. Q: Yes, my mother was always complaining about being sick, and I always had to try to calm her down. It was very annoying. I never wanted to expose my daughter to that.

Th: Well, perhaps you've gone too far in never discussing your problems with her. Then you get angry when she doesn't ask about them.

Ms. Q: Yes. Maybe so. Maybe we can write down your suggestions. I want to go over them before I talk to her.

Th: I think that would be a good idea.

As in Chapter 5 ("A Framework for Targeting Behavioral Change"), writing down behavioral alternatives, along with fears of enacting them and anticipated responses of others, can be valuable as a form of homework in pursuing behavioral change. This approach is particularly helpful in patients who "disconnect," an unconscious form of dissociation to avoid distress created by addressing problems or the response of others. Writing down scripts and monitoring their use and avoidance provide a means for patients to "keep in mind" behavioral alternatives that they quickly forget.

### Case Example

Ms. I (see Chapters 4 and 5) would regularly have "brain freeze," as she named it, when she intended to confront others about difficult topics. Thus, she would tend not to recall particular scripts when it was time to express them and sometimes struggled to remember them moments after they were discussed in a session. In these circumstances, the therapist can work both to identify what is triggering the problem with recall and review the scripts, possibly having the patient write them down. In the case of Ms. I, the therapist and patient had discussed in the previous session wanting to suggest couples therapy to her husband and a particular script for doing so.

> Ms. I: Now I don't even remember what to say about why I wanted couples' therapy.
> Therapist: What do you think happened? You were just describing last session about what it would be like to talk with Tom about it, as well as your frustrations and fears of hurting him.
> Ms. I: I don't know, but I'm beginning to recognize that this is what happens to me. It's what we talked about as brain freeze. I know we were talking about couples therapy and it made sense to me, but I don't recall what we were saying.
> Th: So I wonder if being on the verge of actually speaking to him frightened you.
> Ms. I: That could be true. Once I plan to talk to him all my worries come to the fore. Like how he will attack me and it won't go anywhere.
> Th: Well, we had discussed your saying, "I think we have problems communicating about issues because we get into a fight. I think we need someone to help us."
> Ms. I: You know, I'm going to write these things down. I think it helps me when I start to disconnect. (Patient takes out a pen and paper and begins writing.) Also what he'll say and what I might say. Because as soon as he begins to get angry with me, I just completely lose what I'm saying.
> Th: I think that it's important that we anticipate how he tends to respond, what happens with your feelings, and how you might respond back.
> Ms. I: So if I say couples therapy would help with our fighting, Tom's going to say, "What do you mean fight? We're not having a fight," or, "You're making me anxious." Or he'll say, "Oh, you just want to get rid of me." And I think part of me does want to end the relationship. And then I'm stumped. I'll write those down as well.

Th: Okay. What's happening to you inside at that point?

Ms. I: I'm just frustrated and anxious. But I lose it then. That's when I disconnect.

Th: I think we need to explore more about what happens at this point. But I think you can say that he's giving a perfect example of the problem if he dismisses what you say. Or if he says, "You're trying to get rid of me," you can say, "No I'm not. That's why I want couples therapy." If he says, "You're making me anxious," you can say, "Well, that's why we need help communicating better."

Ms. I: Those responses make sense. Maybe writing them down will help me remember them better. Although at other times I do confront him more than I did before. I guess I need to understand more why I suddenly shut down.

Th: I think certain topics have become safer for you. In certain instances you feel safer to speak, whereas with others you reflexively shut down.

As indicated above, when identifying behavioral scripts, the psychodynamic therapist will typically address and explore interfering factors as well. In the following vignette the therapist indicates how Ms. B's behavioral struggles (see Chapters 2 and 6) lead her to consider expressing her feelings in a way that increases her guilt and intrapsychic conflict. The suggested alternative, which is less critical, is more acceptable to the patient.

### Case Example

Although Ms. B felt safer overall with her fiancé than with her mother and aunt, she occasionally had difficulties addressing problems with him. Ms. B described how she was having difficulty with her fiancé's unwillingness to participate in social activities, frustrated with the limitations it placed on their social life. In part, working with her efforts to assert her own needs, she pushed him to get together more often with their friends, and things had improved. However, he wanted considerable positive feedback about participating and afterward complained that he was exhausted and needed her to take on more chores. Ms. B struggled with understanding and empathizing with his social anxieties on the one hand and being annoyed with his expectations on the other.

Ms. B: I get mad and I want to say to Jim, "You need to grow up and face getting together with my friends. That's just what adults do." But I know that's kind of harsh and I feel guilty about it.

*Identifying Alternative Behaviors*

> Therapist: It seems like you have trouble recognizing that you can both have empathy for his situation and be frustrated with him. You can be understanding about his anxiety and furious with him about his difficulties being social and his subsequent demands.
>
> Ms. B: That makes sense, but it's very irritating about how much positive feedback he wants for doing these activities. He's joking a bit, but then he really does expect me to do more chores.
>
> Th: Well, one option would be to joke with him about it. "Okay let's see how many compliments you require or how many tasks I have to do. I'd like to see if we could cut down a bit on that."
>
> Ms. B: He might think that's funny, but I get stuck because I'm so mad. When I was a kid and my brother and I were shy, my mother would just push us in front of people. She would say, "Just deal with it."
>
> Th: I think that might be part of the source of your struggle confronting him. Although you think your mother had a point, I think you also don't want to be harsh in the way she was because that felt very uncaring to you.
>
> Ms. B: Yeah, it does sound similar to what I was thinking of saying to him. I didn't realize that.
>
> Th: I think if you consider ways of addressing Jim that don't feel so angry it would be easier to confront him. We could discuss other ideas for doing this if you don't like the humorous approach I suggested.
>
> Ms. B: I can try to do that. We'll see how it goes.

Here the intensity of Ms. B's angry fantasies interfered with behavioral steps to address areas of tension with Jim. Her irritation can be in part derived from a build-up of frustration from not dealing with problems over time. This intensification can cause the anger to emerge in fantasies or behavior in which the patient behaves in unempathic, critical, or other hurtful ways, triggering anxiety and guilt. This pattern is common in patients like Ms. B, when parents have not aided children in developing skills to address and negotiate their needs or were critical or intrusive in their demands of their children.

Ms. B's struggle with identification with the aggressor added to her internal struggles. In this defense (described in Chapter 4) patients link themselves, often unconsciously, with someone who has had power or control over them and used it in damaging and hurtful ways. This identification is accompanied by fantasies of treating others in the way that they were treated when vulnerable and can help them to feel in control at least initially. However, the defense can trigger intense guilty feelings about inflicting pain that the patients themselves experienced. Thus the therapist gently reminds Ms. B that she had described her mother's behavior toward her when she was shy as very hurtful, and she was likely experiencing considerable guilt when she considered expressing "harsh" attitudes toward her fiancé.

Another valuable tool alluded to in these vignettes is the use of humor in behavioral interventions. Humor is considered a high-level defense, as it is often employed to address uncomfortable or conflicted topics indirectly. A current example would be the broad range of explicit sexual humor in television sitcoms regarding topics previously considered as taboo. As such, humor can often be used to indirectly address areas of tension in interpersonal and couples' relationships. Not all individuals are comfortable using humor and not all are capable of accepting it, but the therapist can suggest some possibilities and see how patients and their partners or friends respond. Also, sometimes patients independently use humor in these circumstances; the therapist can note how it was employed and discuss its potential in other circumstances.

> As Ms. B began to more comfortably consider the dynamics involved in these tensions with Jim, she realized how she was agreeing to do things that he wanted her to do with his family, while he balked at similar activities with hers. In this case the therapist used the patient's suggested behavioral alternative as a basis to confront her about conflicted feelings in asserting her needs.

> Ms. B: So then Jim said, "I don't want to go to breakfast with your family. We just had dinner with them." But I was annoyed because I spend a lot of time with his family on vacations, and I don't always want to do it.
> Th: I think it's certainly okay when visiting in-laws or even one's own family to take breaks. I guess you're worried about asking for breaks from his family.
> Ms. B: That's true. I feel like I do everything with them. It's just kind of expected and I'm resentful about it.
> Th: Have you spoken to him about it?
> Ms. B: No. I'm just doing what I think I'm supposed to do. And then it seems unfair he gets out of spending time with my family or other activities because of his anxiety. Maybe I should talk to him. But then I feel selfish.
> Th: Well, what would you say to him?

Ms. B: I would say, "I don't see why I have to spend all the time with your family when we get together but you don't have to do the same with my family. I would like to take some breaks too."

Th: Well, hearing what you might say, I'm not sure what's selfish about it. I certainly think it's okay to say that you should both be able to take family breaks. It sounds like being selfish is the equivalent of expressing any of your own wishes, which we know causes you discomfort.

Ms. B: I guess I'm just being the good girl again. I better discuss that with him.

The identification of behavioral alternatives provides a pathway for patients to more directly confront their intrapsychic and interpersonal fears. Examination of these fears provides additional information about patients' psychodynamics at the same time that it opens up a process of experimentation with new behavioral paradigms. As will be discussed in the following chapters, the therapist works collaboratively with the patient in examining the outcomes of patients' behavioral efforts and adjusting their behaviors accordingly.

# 8

# Identifying Interfering Factors in Performing Alternative Behaviors

Once alternative behaviors are identified, it can take considerable therapeutic work for patients to implement these changes in a consistent way. To aid in this process, the therapist and patient can examine what interferes with moving forward with the behavior. Despite intending to pursue a new course of action (or holding back from an action), the patient may forget about the alternative in the relevant circumstances or consider the alternative but not perform it. If the patient does not think of implementing the behavioral change, the therapist can explore why the alternative did not come to mind. The patient may be repressing or denying the potential change because of various feelings or conflicts, which can be explored in that context. If the patient considers but hesitates making the behavioral change, the therapist and patient can examine the emotions and fantasies occurring at that time. In this way, the identification of alternative behaviors can be used as a tool to determine interfering feelings and conflicts that inhibit implementation and to develop new strategies that address these factors (Table 8–1). These aspects frequently emerge and can be explored in the transference, as the patient can have a variety of reactions to the therapist when considering behaviors that may feel awkward or scary.

## Monitoring Thoughts and Feelings

The development of self-observational capacity was discussed in Chapter 5, "A Framework for Targeting Behavioral Change." In these circumstances the therapist and patient apply these approaches with regard to consideration of a specific behavior. Homework, discussed below, can also be useful in monitoring and addressing factors that interfere with an intended behavioral change.

## Identifying Specific Interfering Factors

Many forms of resistance can occur in response to considering implementing a behavioral change. They include various forms of intrapsychic conflicts, defenses, fantasies, and self and object representations, and this chapter describes some of these factors (see Table 8–1). For example, if the change involves increased assertiveness, patients may link the behavior to angry or competitive feelings, or increased autonomy, which can create fears of damaging and disrupting relationships. The association of effective changes with aggressive feelings and fantasies can trigger guilt and a felt need for self-punishment. Patients may feel inadequate or incapable of making a change and could potentially be concerned about disappointing the therapist. As noted in Chapter 3 ("Identifying and Addressing Risks in Targeting Behavioral Change"), direct targeting of behavioral change can trigger a rebellious or anxious response when the patient internally sees it as being imposed on them, sometimes viewing the therapist as a frightening and commanding authority.

### Struggles With Assertiveness

In assessing factors that interfere with taking behavioral steps, a particular action can be identified as a goal. In a patient who struggles with assertiveness, these behaviors will typically involve addressing an issue with an important person in the patient's life. The identification of this specific action allows for a closer examination of various fantasies, feelings, and conflicts that are inhibitory, promoting the analytic process. Interfering factors often include anxiety about potentially disrupting the relationship or provoking rejection, or guilt about possibly damaging the

**TABLE 8–1.** Identifying factors interfering with performing alternative behaviors

Monitoring thoughts and feelings as behavior is considered
Identifying specific interfering factors
    Struggles with fears of assertiveness
    Feelings of inadequacy
    Rebellious reactions
Using homework to identify and address interfering factors

other person. As in the case below, first discussed in Chapter 4 ("Using Psychodynamic Techniques in Addressing Behavioral Change") and then continued in Chapters 5 and 7 ("Identifying Alternative Behaviors"), this exploration can also lead to a modification of the planned action.

### Case Example

The therapist and Ms. I had identified behavioral goals that included greater assertion of her needs. To better implement these behaviors, they focused on a particular difficulty, getting her husband to seek medical evaluation of his somatic complaints. Ms. I wondered whether these symptoms represented anxiety or depression rather than a medical disorder. In spite of experiencing significant distress, Tom was resistant to seeing a doctor. He would sometimes agree to go but then not follow through. Ms. I had addressed this pattern with him, but he became frustrated in response. In addition to his suffering, Tom was more rigid and critical of Ms. I when he was experiencing somatic distress. After identifying the adverse impact on her, she and the therapist were able to examine struggles she had being definitive about his need for help. They discussed how it was important for her to insist on his seeing a doctor. Ms. I seemed to feel that the only option that would change Tom's mind was to threaten to end the relationship, but she was frightened that he might reject her in response. The therapist explored why she saw addressing this issue as an ultimatum.

> Ms. I: I feel that I'm saying to him that if he doesn't do it, the relationship will be over. If I give him an ultimatum I think it will be very hurtful for him. I don't think I can do that.
> Therapist: Well, I'm not sure I understand why it has to be an ultimatum in which you directly threaten the relationship. Why can't you just say that he has to get treatment, that his

anxiety creates a lot of pain for you and him. Why do you feel this would disrupt the relationship?

Ms. I: That's an interesting way of saying it. I'll consider it. I do think of my father when I think how it might hurt him. I also worry that even if I put it that way, Tom will think that I'm threatening to end the relationship. And then I get worried that he'll try to end it.

Th: Has he ever actually threatened this?

Ms. I: No.

Th: Then I think that this idea really stems from your own fears. Or maybe you could have a wish he would end the relationship?

Ms. I: Well, I don't think so, but it could be. Then it wouldn't be my responsibility.

After acknowledging that it did not need to be presented as an ultimatum, Ms. I increased her efforts but still struggled to be firm, and exploration revealed additional conflicts.

Ms. I: I still can't make him go to the doctor. It's always like, "I'll go when I feel better." I get furious at him. That's when I have "brain freeze." I forget what we discussed saying to him.

Th: Well, we can certainly review what you might say, and writing it down may be helpful. What do you think happens when you have "brain freeze"?

Ms. I: I worry I'm going to hurt him. That I'll lose control.

Th: What would losing control look like?

Ms. I: I'm not sure. Maybe I would start screaming and cursing at him.

Th: I think you get really frightened of your anger because you feel you will lose control like your father and sister did. Then there will just always be fighting with no solutions.

Ms. I: You know it's funny you should say that. Because the other day I had the thought, "Now I see how a wife could punch a husband." Then I felt terrible and guilty. If I did that I could end up in jail!

Th: I think it's good you're aware of those thoughts because they may be a missing link in what frightens you so much. You can be clear now that that's just an expression of how strongly you feel and nothing you would really do.

Ms. I: Sometimes I feel like I could act on my anger, but I know I wouldn't. It's interesting. The other day I was furious at my associate. I started to get anxious about being mean and began to lose my nerve. But then I recognized that as his

> boss I needed to address the problem. When I said something then I calmed down.
>
> Th: Once you see that your anger will not be out of control, you're less anxious. That's important that you were able to take that step with your associate. Maybe you could think about how effective this was when you try to address problems with your husband.
>
> Ms. I: Okay, well, now I think I'd really be able to do it.

## Feelings of Inadequacy

Feelings of inadequacy and an anticipated inability to accomplish a task often interfere with taking steps to achieve behavioral change. Sometimes patients are actually not capable of performing a particular action and some additional training may be required. At other points patients may not know how to go about addressing a specific problem. In these instances, discussions about particular types of interventions can be of value, as was discussed in Chapter 7 ("Identifying Alternative Behaviors"). In other situations, patients struggle with fantasies of inadequacy, and they are indeed capable of enacting a behavior. These fantasies should be addressed, along with conflicts and feelings that may be contributory to this self-perception. For example, patients with assertiveness fears may have a fantasy of inadequacy to protect against conflicted angry feelings associated with a sense of empowerment. These factors contributed to Mr. E's (see Chapters 3 and 6) struggles about completing his consulting work:

> Mr. E: I know I'm supposed to do this work, but I'm just not doing it. I'm putting if off. And then I just feel guilty and lazy.
>
> Therapist: Let's talk about what you feel when you sit down to do it.
>
> Mr. E: I just feel like I'm not capable of doing it. I think that the guy I'm consulting for is sitting there thinking that I'm terrible at this, even though he asked me to do the job.
>
> Th: Well, what is it you need to do?
>
> Mr. E: I need to get some information from a colleague of mine. He's happy to provide it, but so far I haven't even sent the request. Then I have to organize a chart for what factors to look at.
>
> Th: So are you actually capable of doing this work?
>
> Mr. E: Well…yes, I can do it.
>
> Th: So that's important that you feel incapable but actually can do the work. We need to understand more about this fantasy.
>
> Mr. E: I just say I'm going to look up this one thing on the Internet and then get to it, but then I never get back to it. And my wife, as you

might expect, is really pushing me to do it. She's saying I'm lazy. And I get angry about that, but I feel guilty too.

Th: I think we've come to understand that your wife is providing the punishment for you that part of you thinks is appropriate. Because you feel guilty and lazy. But your anger raises another question: Is this part of your feeling angry about having to work?

Mr. E: I know we've talked about my anger. That I feel I should just be taken care of and that it's not fair.

Th: Yes, like when you were a kid and your mother moved with you to a new home after the divorce. You were angry about the change and thought what's the point of making any effort? Kind of a sit-down strike.

Mr. E: I see what you're saying. But what's more accessible to me is not feeling capable.

Th: And yet you've said that in fact you could do this work. I think that perhaps seeing yourself as incompetent protects you against fears of your anger. At the same time you indirectly express it by not doing the work you feel others are pressuring you to do.

Mr. E: Well, that makes sense. But how can I stop doing this?

Th: Okay. Well I think you should consider setting specific times for doing the work. Be alert that you're going to feel an urge to do other things and see if you can steer yourself back to the work. If you feel incapable I think you need to question this notion. I think you should also try to access any anger you might feel at that point. It's important to be aware that avoiding the work leads to your feeling more undermined.

Mr. E: Okay. That's helpful.

## Rebellious Reactions to Behavioral Change

As noted above, patients may view a behavioral change as a threat to their self-esteem, or as pressure from the therapist and others, against which they rebel. Identifying this resistance is important, as it is often hidden from view and can be explored within the context of the transference.

In the following vignette the therapist addresses Mr. G's (see Chapter 3) feelings of anger and injury in response to others, including the therapist, who encourage him to search for a job.

### Case Example

Despite Mr. G's stated intent, and growing financial difficulties, the patient continued to make very little effort in his job search. Work in the transference helped the patient to recognize that he expected the therapist to be an unthinking authority rather than someone trying to help him. The therapist differentiated himself from an unempathic authority, stating that he was deeply concerned about the patient's feelings and his struggles. The therapist encouraged him to set aside time for a job search, observing what interfered with his pursuing this.

> Mr. G: I get very upset when I start to search for jobs. I see an ad for a barista, and then I think, there's no way I'm going to work at a coffee shop. I wouldn't be able to tolerate it.
>
> Therapist: From what we've talked about before you want to pursue your writing, but you feel frustrated and disappointed that it's hard to make money in this. You don't want to have a job that other people have, because you want to feel special; it's a blow to your self-esteem. So you avoid looking for a job because that would make you like everyone else.
>
> Mr. G: Okay. So I know that, but I still don't look for a job. What am I supposed to do about that?
>
> Th: I think that even asking me that question is a form of avoidance. You might even be mad at me for wanting you to look at the feelings preventing your job search. Because you're angry about considering it. You said if other therapists started to push you too much to make changes you let them know you didn't want to do it.
>
> Mr. G: Yes. Well that's true, but it still doesn't help me look.
>
> Th: I think that's because you're making a conscious decision not to look at your behavior more directly because it's too painful. You said the other day you had the thought that you could look for a job, but then what happened? That's what we need to look at.
>
> Mr. G: Well, I don't even remember what happened. I guess as I thought about specific jobs I could look into I lost all my energy. I just went to watch TV.
>
> Th: You must have shut that down inside very quickly.
>
> Mr. G: Yeah. I guess I did. Like I said, it would feel terrible to me. I would feel like a prisoner who is being punished. I guess I am mad at you. You feel more like a jailer than a therapist. On the other hand, I know that you're doing your job.
>
> Th: I think we need to look at that sense of me as a jailer and your being imprisoned and understand it better. Obviously that adds to your difficulties in the job search and in therapy. But it is catastrophic thinking: a job isn't a prison.
>
> Mr. G: Okay, but it feels that way. And I also hope something or someone will save me from this fate. The cavalry will come over the hill and maybe I'll get to stick with my writing.

In addition to feeling narcissistically injured pursuing a job inconsistent with his career goals and self-view, Mr. G hoped, often unconsciously, that he would be rescued from needing a job he did not want. When he was young, he was halfhearted about math and science homework, and his family often signaled that this was not a problem, believing he should focus on his creative writing, in which he showed early promise. When Mr. G got into trouble with his grades, his father would "rescue" him, spending a significant amount of time on his homework. Despite his father no longer being actively involved in his affairs, Mr. G continued to have magical fantasies of rescue that affected his job search.

Mr. G: I don't feel I need to get a job where I feel demeaned.
Th: What do you imagine would happen if you run out of money?
Mr. G: I feel someone will come in and rescue me. I wouldn't end up out on the street.
Th: Who do you feel would do this?
Mr. G: My father. Like he always used to do with my homework. Or maybe something would come through and I'll get a regular writing job.
Th: Is your father in a position to rescue you now?
Mr. G: I actually think he couldn't financially handle it right now.
Th: So this really represents a fantasy that you'll be rescued, based on what you experienced in your childhood.
Mr. G: Yes. I really feel strongly that it will happen. Maybe because it happened so many times.
Th: I think this may be significantly inhibiting your job search. We really need to address the power of this fantasy. Maybe you're mad that I can't rescue you from your predicament.
Mr. G: Well, yes, I do feel mad that I'm still struggling with this and you're not helping me more. But I also realize that there are limitations in what you can do. You can't get me a job.

## Using Homework

As discussed in Chapter 5, there are several forms of homework that may be valuable in psychodynamic psychotherapy targeting behavioral problems. A diary can be used to track thoughts, feelings, and symptoms that arise in the context of attempting to accomplish a particular behavior. This information helps to identify interferences with accomplishing the alternative behavior, such as particular conflicts, defenses, and fantasies. Often these fantasies and feelings have escaped patients' awareness or not emerged in therapy because they are painful for patients to consider, and writing them down may increase conscious access. Furthermore, a diary can aid in the discussion of strategies to counter interfering factors at the point of attempting the behavior. It can be particularly useful for patients who dissociate in these contexts, such as Ms. I. In her case, making notes of her thoughts and feelings helped to identify that the "brain freeze" occurred at the point that she feared losing control of her anger and damaging others.

Patients can also make notes of certain potential scripts, including what they anticipate the response of others will be, what interferes with enacting these scripts, and what their response and that of others is to the actual use of the script. Thus, patients can keep in mind and report to the therapist the impact and experience of their work on particular behavioral interventions. As can be noted in the case examples in this chapter, addressing fears and interfering factors about performing a behavior can aid in the working through process. As contributors to inhibiting changes are identified over time, new interventions can be formulated. As demonstrated below, homework can aid in this working through process.

### Case Example: Ms. I (*continued*)

Ms. I continued to struggle with addressing her concerns with her husband. Writing down the series of problems, comments, and anticipated responses aided her in avoiding "brain freeze." Using a diary in which she kept track of her thoughts, the therapist and she identified more clearly a series of factors as she considered making her comments to Tom. These included a fear that he would feel rejected by her, causing him intense distress. A second worry was that he would reject her if she confronted him about problems. However, her husband had never made any comments about leaving her, only fears of her rejecting him. And a third fear was that if she asked him to make changes and he was not able to do so, then she would end up rejecting him. Using this information the therapist was able to directly address each of her anxieties. He pointed out that she might feel better about the relationship in general if she expressed her concerns to Tom and may not feel any wish to end the relationship. Second, even if he was unable to make changes, she did not have to reject him. Third, if he struggled with making changes, she could further press him to seek psychotherapy, which she wanted him to pursue in any case. For example, she felt therapy would better help him to manage his anxiety, which contributed to his attempts to control her.

Ms. I discussed her difficulty confronting her associate about not completing tasks that she expected of him. Again she identified "brain freeze," noting that his response would upend her. The therapist suggested that she write down her possible responses, as she did with her husband. A written record would help keep these ideas in mind and diminish her tendency to disconnect.

>Therapist: What do you anticipate he'll say?
>Ms. I: Well, if I say you're not fulfilling your role in this position, he'll say, "Well you haven't supported me in this position." Then I'm not sure what to say to that.
>Th: Well, you could just say you see it differently.
>Ms. I: I just get stuck and I don't say it.
>Th: I think it's because you view any direct discussion of your frustration as catastrophically damaging to the other person and the relationship. Then you have brain freeze and don't say it.
>Ms. I: That's true, but how can I remember?
>Th: By continuing to help you identify that it's not catastrophic. It's just a typical thing a boss would say. But I also think it might be helpful to write it down. That seems to help you keep these comments in mind.
>Ms. I: Yes, and maybe it would help to write down what I see as dangerous about them.

# 9

# Working With Sustaining Behavioral Change and the Response of Others

The therapist and patient work in an ongoing way to assess the degree of behavioral change and its impact on the patient's self-perceptions, fantasies, emotions, conflicts, and interpersonal relationships (Table 9–1). Although patients usually develop a heightened sense of empowerment, less severe intrapsychic conflict, less intense negative affects, and improved relationships with behavioral change, guilty or anxious reactions can also occur. Additionally, problematic behavior, although improved, can persist in certain circumstances or may recur. In psychodynamic psychotherapy, these incidences can be viewed as opportunities for ongoing addressing of conflicts, dynamics, and behavior as part of the working through process. Attending to these factors is important for generalizing and sustaining changes. Another potential area of difficulty is an inadequate or adverse response from others to behavioral changes. The patient needs to address these responses, either in continued efforts to change the other person's behavior, an acceptance of that behavior, a modification of the relationship, or a search for new relationships. Unexpected problematic reactions by others may lead to a reassessment of approaches and potential work in the transference, depending on the patient's reaction (e.g., blaming the therapist).

## Addressing Intrapsychic Conflicts and Negative Affects From Behavioral Change

Behavioral changes that have occurred in the course of therapy are generally experienced positively but can trigger intrapsychic conflicts and guilty or anxious reactions. Patients may need to adjust to perceptions of themselves as more effective. They may also be fearful that the changes have damaged or hurt others, or may lead to retaliation, even as they experience beneficial responses. Patients may unconsciously enact self-punitive behaviors or draw back from new changes. Freud (1916/1957) referred to a group of patients "wrecked by success" who felt guilty about favorable changes in their lives and unconsciously became self-destructive in response. Such internal conflicts and guilt and anxiety need to be addressed for patients to continue to move forward with and sustain the changes they are making. When others are reacting positively, contrasting the patient's guilt and anxiety with these responses can be helpful.

### Case Example

Mr. T, a 46-year-old salesman at a tech company, began to be more assertive at his work through his treatment and was able to land an important client for his company. However, following this achievement he was beset by guilt and anxiety, fearing that he had hurt and angered his colleagues or triggered retaliation from his boss. Exploration of his past history had identified Mr. T's experience of a bullying father as an inhibitor of more assertive behavior. He anticipated his bosses and others at his work as potentially reacting like his father, becoming punitive to demonstrate they were in control and could not tolerate someone else having power. Understanding these factors had aided him in becoming bolder at work, helping him to get the new client.

> Therapist: So what makes you think you have caused so much damage and will get in trouble. This is what they want you to do at the company, right?
> Mr. T: Well it's very competitive there, and I think some of my colleagues are going to be jealous. They announce these things at the Friday meeting.
> Th: Well, I understand that, but how is this different from competitive environments at any workplace? You seem to believe

**TABLE 9–1.** Working with the degree and impact of behavioral change

Addressing intrapsychic conflict and negative emotions generated by behavioral change

Dealing with behavioral change that does not generalize

Addressing recurrence of problematic behavior

Dealing with the response of others to behavioral change

---

the impact will be much more negative than usually happens in these circumstances.

Mr. T: Yes, that's true. And I also think my boss is going to be mad. I know that sounds strange, but I think he'll see me as "getting too big for my britches."

Th: What do you think he'll do?

Mr. T: Reprimand me, maybe for being too aggressive in pursuing the client.

Th: Doesn't it benefit him when you get more work? It sounds a lot like your fears with your father, that he couldn't really tolerate you having your own ideas and successes.

Mr. T: That's true. I even got worried you would get mad. That somehow you would feel threatened by me.

Th: I guess it's hard to believe that I would want you to feel more empowered, based on your experiences.

Mr. T: I guess I'm not used to it.

The therapist and patient came to recognize that although he had felt safer in his efforts to seek new clients, signing this significant one somehow "crossed a line." Identifying his fears and the lack of the anticipated adverse reactions from others eased his guilt and anxiety, and he felt safer continuing to assert himself more in the work setting.

# Dealing With Behavioral Change That Does Not Generalize

Behavioral change in a particular circumstance does not necessarily generalize to other related situations, because the contributory fears and conflicts are broadly ingrained and/or because the different circumstances generate different dynamics and emotions. For instance, Mr. C (see Chapter 3, "Identifying and Addressing Risks in Targeting Behavioral Change") was able to be more assertive with his boss but still felt unable to confront the demeaning comments of his girlfriend. To highlight this predicament, the therapist might say, "We know you made these changes from how you behave now with person A or circumstance B, and we need to understand why this other situation is more difficult." Identification and exploration of this variability will help broaden understanding of the patient's dynamics and aid in adjusting behavioral interventions, another aspect of the working through process. This knowledge will also help to expand the behaviors to additional situations in which change has not occurred. In Mr. T's case, examining inhibitions with a colleague after successfully overcoming them in some circumstances aided in the identification of a new relevant dynamic.

### Case Example: Mr. T (*continued*)

Mr. T: So I know our discussion was helpful to me. I was able to overcome my fears and call Dev, and he definitely wanted to hire me as a consultant. And I think, "Why didn't I call him sooner?"

Th: Based on your father's critical and bullying attitudes we understand part of why you mistakenly expected Dev to reject you. As you consider other business opportunities, we should remember how this colleague's response was so positive.

Mr. T: Yes, that's a good idea. Because I notice that I need to make some more calls and I'm still fearful about some of them.

Th: Okay, well, why don't we talk about a specific person you're hesitating calling and see what you might be avoiding.

Mr. T: Okay, well there's Eric. I think it's interesting because he's actually a colleague in a competing position. So I really don't know whether he's going to help. But I thought of a way we might be able to work together to get more business. I guess if he doesn't want to he'll just say no.

Th: So what are you worried about?

Mr. T: Well, I was imagining he would say, "Are you kidding, no one would ever give you that business. They know you're not competent." But now that I think about it, there's no reason for him to say that. Either he'll want to collaborate or he won't.

Th: So again, you seem to be expecting negative responses based on your past. But maybe you find competitive feelings particularly threatening?

> Mr. T: I think I'm worried about his being competitive with me. But I think I also feel competitive with him, and I'm not sure I'm comfortable with that. We would be working together, but the person that signs a particular client gets higher share of the money.
> Th: What do you think the problem is with feeling competitive?
> Mr. T: Well, I get kind of stirred up when I'm competing. Maybe I could get mean. I might try to shut him out of certain negotiations.
> Th: Okay, well, that's definitely something to explore further. Let's find out more about how you would be mean. Maybe you're worried you'll become bullying like your father?
> Mr. T: Maybe.

Work on Mr. T's rejection fears had focused on his expectation that others would reject him. However, as he felt safer he began to identify his own competitive urges and fears that he would be mean like his father if he had power, an example of identification with the aggressor (see Chapter 11, "Addressing Behavioral Problems Related to Adverse Developmental Experiences and Trauma"). This new dynamic was another previously unrecognized contributor to his inhibitions.

As noted above, addressing one contributory factor with resulting behavioral change may lead to another becoming more accessible.

### Case Example

Mr. U, a 64-year-old business executive, had made headway in addressing fears of confronting his friend, whom he had tended to see as a critical authority reminiscent of his temperamental father, but still had difficulty asserting himself with his wife. In this instance, identifying a previously undiscussed developmental experience aided in recognizing why fears of his wife persisted.

> Mr. U: I'm upset I'm still having trouble confronting Linda.
> Therapist: Well, it's interesting because we know you've made headway with Rob but still struggle with her. We want to understand why that is.
> Mr. U: That's true. I still find it to be very scary.
> Th: Well, we know you were scared with Rob and now it doesn't even bother you to talk to him about problems. So something that stopped being a fear with him is still an issue with your wife. We identified part of it as connected with Rob's temper, which reminded you of your father.

Mr. U: I feel I could be more direct with her; I've been able to confront her at times, but it's tough. But you reminded me of something. When my father didn't like something, sometimes he would start yelling. But other times he wouldn't talk to me for days, and in some ways that was worse. And not only that: my mom would go along with him! She would withdraw rather than be her usual caring self.

Th: So how do you think that may affect your greater fears with your wife?

Mr. U: Well, I'm around her more of the time, so it's going to have more impact on me if she gets upset. And come to think of it, she does get silent when she's mad. That's very upsetting to me and it was when I was a kid.

Th: We should definitely talk more about the silences. They sound very frightening to you. But when you have confronted her, her angry withdrawal has been very brief. Not as you expected.

Mr. U: That's true. Well, this may help me to try it more with her.

# Addressing Recurrence of Problematic Behavior

In many instances, patients suffer a setback or recurrence with a behavior that they had made headway in changing. This is not surprising given that many behaviors are habitual and occur almost reflexively under certain conditions. Also, a more intense experience of feelings and conflicts may have emerged in the context of particular circumstances or stressors, triggering the behaviors. The therapist should reassure the patient that this is not unusual and that sustaining behavior requires continued efforts to observe and intervene with contributors. At other times this recurrence suggests that additional dynamics and developmental events have not been addressed, and the therapist and patient should attempt to identify them.

### Case Example: Mr. U (*continued*)

At a later point Mr. U had a sudden resurgence of anxiety and inhibition with his friend Rob, after he had made significant progress in asserting himself in their relationship.

Th: So tell me about what happened?

Mr. U: Well, Rob had important information about when a business deal would be completed. So I asked him what it was.

And he refused to tell me, saying that he had promised the person who told him that he wouldn't tell anybody! He's always shared information with me and he knows I keep confidences. I felt furious and dumbfounded, but I couldn't think of anything to say. I mean what is this, second grade? I won't tell him how angry I am.

Th: It sounds like you already have some ideas about what you might say. But what are you worried is going to happen if you do confront him?

Mr. U: I'm scared of his anger. I don't want him to get mad or stop talking to me. Like my father.

Th: Well, I know that hasn't happened since you've been more assertive with Rob. I wonder if this time you're worried because you're so enraged with him.

Mr. U: Well that's right. I mean I can't believe he said that. He knows how I never tell anyone any secret. So it's insulting. But I'm worried about telling him how angry I am. Even though I haven't set him off that could do it.

Th: Well, I'm not sure it would. But maybe you could just tell him you feel hurt and insulted. And also, wouldn't it help your getting the business deal done if you have this information?

Mr. U: Definitely, and I'll need to let him know that. But you're right. Maybe telling him I'm hurt and not directly saying I'm angry will help. It certainly makes me feel safer. I notice my fear of talking to him has suddenly eased.

In this instance Mr. U's more intense anger triggered anxiety and a resurgence of conflicts, increasing his defensive avoidance. As with many individuals with a temperamental parent, he needed to recognize that his anger could be used in more effective ways. Additional therapeutic work was necessary to help him to tolerate these rageful feelings, allowing him to sustain his assertive behavior.

# Dealing With the Response of Others to Behavioral Change

When a patient makes changes in behavior, others often respond in positive ways or accept the new limits. However, some family members, partners, or friends may not react to the new behavior as the patient hoped. They may become angry, ignore the patient's efforts, or simply not make changes. The patient has several options at this point, including the following: continue to address the problem, accept the lack of responsiveness, encourage the other person to seek therapy, enter couples therapy, pull back from the relationship, and/or find new relationships. The patient and therapist must also recognize that response from others is often not immediate, may be inconsistent, or require several efforts. The therapist will assist the patient in continuing to explore whether the patient is inhibited about more forcefully addressing the problem or identify additional alternative strategies.

If there continues to be a lack of response, the patient may need to accept or mourn the shortcomings of a more problematic relationship. Sometimes this process can be difficult because patients must work through feelings of anger or loss. They may have held on to the hope of change despite severe persistent problems. For instance, when a patient attempts to set limits with family members, they may still not be able to respond to these limits, creating frustration and disappointment. The patient may decide to find other ways to curb his or her exposure to these circumstances. Alternatively, the other person may respond to limit setting, but a wished-for increased closeness may not occur. The patient may need to accept these limitations and seek more intimate or responsive relationships outside the family.

As Ms. F (see Chapters 3, 6, and 7) made headway in setting limits with her son, she realized that she also yielded to mistreatment by some of her friends, based on dynamics that were similar to those involving her son. As she recognized this pattern, she began to restrict her contact with them. In the following vignette, Ms. F became frightened about her shrinking social circle, in an interim period when she was looking for new relationships with others who were more responsive.

### Case Example

Ms. F: Now that I've set more limits my social circle has gotten smaller. I noticed that when my friend Jean started to complain to me that I hadn't called her, I really didn't want to have much to do with her, whereas I used to feel I had to apologize. But then I wonder, "Who am I going to get together with?"

Therapist: Well, I guess that's really a consequence of the change in your relationships. They used to be based on your yielding to the needs of others and being very alert to and responsive to their needs. Now you're really not interested in that kind of relationship.

Ms. F: Yes, it's interesting, and I feel better, but I do worry about getting more isolated.

Th: You can meet new friends where there's more give and take in the relationship. Your fear of isolation is probably related to the fear you had as a child that if you didn't respond to your mother's needs you'd be left alone.

Ms. F: Well, that's true. The women I met recently feel much more responsive to what I want. At the same time it's upsetting to feel that I can't be closer to anyone in my family.

Th: That's certainly true. I think it's a loss that you need to mourn further.

Ms. F: I hadn't really thought of it as mourning, but I guess it is mourning of a sort.

As noted earlier in this chapter, sometimes patients may determine that it is best to withdraw from a relationship when others do not respond to their efforts to set limits or promote increased communication. On occasion patients may have trouble withdrawing from a persistently troubled but dramatic and exciting relationship. These relationships can take the form of a sadomasochistic interaction. Part of the inhibition in behavioral change in these circumstances may be not wanting to confront feelings of sadness and loss in giving up the exciting parts of the relationship.

### Case Example

Ms. V, a 28-year-old pharmaceutical sales representative, had been recurrently pulled toward involvements with men who would alternate being close and then suddenly pulling away. She described a background in which there was similar behavior with her mother, who would vary between intense interest in her and periods of withdrawal.

Ms. V: I know my involvement with Juan was troubled, but since I ended my relationship with him I miss the excitement that was involved in it, and I'm kind of sad.

Therapist: Yes, but you kept being pulled into the relationship because he ran hot and cold. And we talked about how it reminded you of your relationship with your mom. You were hoping for a different outcome where you converted him to someone who was consistently loving. But ultimately you would feel disappointed and rejected when he would pull away.

Ms. V: That's absolutely true, but when he was responding to me it was very exciting. I know he was really interested but then he just disconnected. I guess it's just sad that we couldn't work something out. Do you think I'll be able to have that excitement again?

Th: I think we're trying to understand why your excitement gets so intense with someone who does disconnect. As we've understood more about that, recently you have become more interested in men who are more responsive.

Ms. V: Well, there's Michael who's very interested in me and seems like a more responsible guy. It doesn't seem as exciting, but maybe I should give it a chance. I do like him.

# Dealing With Adverse Reactions of Others to Behavioral Change

Sometimes efforts at behavioral change lead to adverse responses that the therapist or patient may have known was a risk or had not anticipated. For instance, if a patient is more assertive, others may react critically or withdraw. The therapist works with the patient to absorb the consequences of this response as with any development in the patient's life. As noted in Chapter 5, "A Framework for Targeting Behavioral Change," it is important for the therapist to let patients know that the outcome of any intervention is uncertain. However, this discussion may be forgotten or overridden by the patient's fantasies about the outcome or the therapist's ability to resolve problems. In these circumstances, patients may blame the therapist for a negative outcome. The therapist may express regret at the result, but this circumstance represents an opportunity to explore the patient's feelings and fantasies in the transference.

### Case Example

Ms. W, a 54-year-old divorced high school science teacher, whose background included tremendous pressure to take care of her anxious mother as well as her younger siblings, struggled with attacks and criticisms by her two younger sisters, which she accepted. She viewed such hostile behavior as fitting punishment for enjoyment of her own intellectual interests, which her siblings did not share. In addition, therapeutic exploration revealed that she felt it was unacceptable that she should have her own needs and wishes. When her sisters criticized her for not doing more to help take care of their children or her mother, even though her caretaking of others was extensive, she believed they must be right about her being "irresponsible." Although the patient did not realize it at first, over time she and her therapist identified her sisters' behavior as bullying. As she began to recognize that these criticisms were unfair and

## Working With Sustaining Behavioral Change

inappropriate, she increasingly understood how she should not be tolerating their hurtful behavior.

At a certain point the patient prepared to tell her siblings that she would no longer accept these attacks. She discussed with the therapist what she intended to say and emphasize as they reviewed alternative options. However, the effort to confront them did not go as she had hoped:

> Ms. W: So I explained everything to them and one sister got furious. She stomped out of the room and sent me an angry note afterward. And what's worse, she told my mother and she called to ask me what I had done. My mother was very judgmental, feeling that I had created problems with the family.
> Therapist: It can take some time for a family to adjust to a new stance. However, even though we hoped that your sisters would be able to accept these new limits, it's possible that they won't and we would have to help you deal with that.
> Ms. W: Somehow I thought we expected that I was going to explain the limits to them and they would just accept them. I didn't anticipate that they would respond so angrily.
> Th: So perhaps you're frustrated with me because you felt I gave the impression things would work out differently?
> Ms. W: Maybe. But the other problem is that I think they're right. I do deserve this and I'm bad somehow.
> Th: So it seems like helping you to assert yourself has led to a backlash with them and inside, putting you back in a place where you feel you don't deserve anything.
> Ms. W: Yes, I do think I deserve this reaction. I'm bad for wanting these changes. I think they're right in how they responded to me.
> Th: I guess that's part of why you're mad at me, because I promoted your assertiveness and efforts to have your needs met, and now you're feeling guilty and reprimanded.

Monitoring his countertransference, the therapist realized he felt guilty and concerned that he had somehow led the patient in a problematic direction. On further consideration, he did not believe he implied that a positive outcome was likely, but understood that the patient believed this. However, the therapist recognized in his guilty reaction that the patient was highly guilt prone and blamed herself and him for her family's angry response. Exploring her criticism was a helpful therapeutic intervention, as it gave the patient an opportunity to safely express her anger toward the therapist. The therapist worked to identify why the patient believed she should feel guilty, rather than view it as a symptom, losing track of the progress she had made. The therapist helped her reconsider that when she was attacked the problem often stemmed from critical reactions and competitive feelings of her sisters rather than her being a "bad" person.

Over the next few weeks the patient emerged from this self-critical state and again recognized her sisters' response was problematic, and her family demonstrated an inability to accept her needs and feelings, part of a longstanding pattern. Around the same time, one of her sisters offered an apology and began to act differently toward Ms. W, being much less critical. Her sister's ultimate response aided further in recognizing that her guilt was excessive, and indeed she was able to change others' attitudes.

This case demonstrates again how behavioral changes led to a revision of the formulation and helped the patient to step back, observe, and repair problematic representations of self and others.

## Reference

Freud S: Some character-types met with in psycho-analytic work (1916), in Standard Edition of the Complete Psychological Works of Sigmund Freud, Vol 14. Translated and edited by Strachey J. London, Hogarth Press, 1957, pp 309–333

# 10

# Engaging the Patient in Addressing Specific Behavioral Problems

This chapter demonstrates how the patient and therapist identify and target common behavioral problems by using the model and approaches described in Chapters 5 through 9. The problems that will be used as examples include conflicts with a partner, difficulty setting limits with children, problems that are identified by others, and difficulties with impulse control (Table 10–1). The therapist develops a formulation based on developmental contributors, fantasies, intrapsychic conflicts, and defenses, and then employs this framework in identifying alternative approaches and addressing factors that inhibit enacting these alternatives (Table 10–2). Finally, the therapist and patient assess and respond to the reactions of others to these changes.

## Marital and Couples' Problems

Marital or couples' problems are a central source of difficulty for many individuals, and most patients demonstrate some degree of adversity in these areas. Patients' core attachment issues and conflicts, as well as disruptions in mentalization, will typically emerge in these intimate relationships. These problems can persist and become more severe over

**TABLE 10–1.** Some common behavioral problems

Marital and couples' problems
Problems with limit setting with children
Problems identified by others
Difficulties with impulse control

---

time, degrading the quality of the relationship. Significant sources of tension include when one member 1) does not express needs and wishes to the other or the other does not respond to or criticizes these needs, or 2) one member accepts behavior that is experienced as problematic, such as persistent attacks, a lack of participation in chores or other responsibilities, or an unresponsiveness to sexual desires. Another common problem is an attack and counterattack pattern with recurrent escalating tensions and fighting. A related problem involves difficulties negotiating differences between partners' needs and wishes. These disagreements can be addressed in couples therapy, but psychodynamic approaches targeting problematic behavioral patterns in individual therapy can often reduce these struggles.

### Case Example

Ms. X, a 48-year-old interior designer, reported a recurrent problematic pattern with her husband. For periods of time they would be close and intimate, with a good sexual relationship. However, he would suddenly withdraw for several weeks, becoming emotionally distant and expressing no sexual interest and little affection. He also became irritable with their two teenage daughters. The patient felt increasingly hurt and frustrated before he finally responded, but would not address the problems with him. The therapist began by exploring her concerns about speaking directly to her husband.

> Therapist: Why don't you talk with him about your frustrations?
> Ms. X: I'm worried he's going to get mad.
> Th: Has this been an issue? It seems like when he gets angry you're able to handle it.
> Ms. X: Well, there is another reason. I'm mad because I don't want to have to be the one to bring it up. That should be his responsibility.
> Th: It sounds like you feel rejected by him in these circumstances.

## TABLE 10–2. Addressing common behavioral problems

Clarifying the specific nature of the problems
Developing a psychodynamic formulation involving contributing factors:
    Developmental contributors
    Self and object representations and associated fantasies
    Intrapsychic conflicts and defenses
    Mentalization difficulties
Identifying specific interventions and alternative approaches based on the formulation
Addressing feelings that inhibit enacting alternative behaviors
Assessing impact of alternative behaviors

---

Ms. X: Yes, I guess. I just assume he's not interested.
Th: But curiously he reengages with you in a loving way after the periods when he's distant.
Ms. X: That's true.
Th: So it's not really clear what's going on with him then. He's also different with the kids, not just you. It might be worth talking to him about it.
Ms. X: Hmm. That's a good point. Well, I'll consider trying it.

However, the patient continued to eschew addressing the issue directly with him, in spite of increasing frustration. The therapist began to explore some possibilities about why Ms. X might be avoiding these discussions, even though she believed it would be a good idea. In exploring her background, she reported a history in which she was close to her father, but felt that her mother was very unresponsive to her or critical when she needed help. Of particular note was when she became very upset about being bullied in junior high school. Her mother did not seem to be interested in what she was contending with and would not talk to her about what to do, despite her entreaties, social isolation, and frequent tearfulness. This experience of a lack of maternal responsiveness repeated itself many times in the patient's life. She had two daughters and made an effort to be available to address their concerns.

The therapist considered that she might be anticipating this pattern with her mother in the relationship with her husband, or was disappointed and frustrated that her husband was not as warmly responsive as her father. The patient found this notion helpful in understanding her feelings, but it had little impact on her sense of being able to talk to her husband. The therapist shifted to exploring what happened as she considered taking a specific action, which provided a further understanding of her inhibitions. As described in Chapter 7 ("Identifying Alternative Behaviors"), he suggested and they discussed possible comments she might make to him, such as, "I don't know if you realize you have this pattern where I feel like you become absent emotionally and you don't want to have sex. Then it's like everything's okay, until it happens again. Are you aware of this?" The therapist employed the approach of being alert to and identifying her feelings and thoughts as she considered speaking to him, asking her to imagine addressing her concerns.

> Th: So what do you fear when you are about to try talking to him, maybe using the comment we discussed?
> Ms. X: I still think he might get mad, but it really feels like he's not going to respond at all. If he ignored me I would get really upset. I'm wrestling already with how mad I am.
> Th: So what about saying that you don't like to be ignored?
> Ms. X: I don't feel like I'm supposed to show those kinds of feelings.
> Th: What comes to mind about that?
> Ms. X: I don't know. You know how I felt with my Mom. How I couldn't get much of a response from her. But when I got older and told her I was mad she was very nasty back. She'd say, "I don't have time for this right now. You'll just have to deal with it."
> Th: I wonder if that's why you assume he won't respond or get furious. That he'll act just like your mother.
> Ms. X: Well, that could be, but right now I'm also worried about how mad I am. I might get really mean and then I'll regret it.
> Th: I recognize that's inhibiting you as well. What would you say?
> Ms. X: I'm not sure. I haven't thought about that really.
> Th: It seems like you worry too much about losing control of your anger. I think we should pay attention to how you might express it. That might help you to be less fearful.

This exchange indicated that the patient experienced conflicts surrounding angry feelings and fantasies and anticipated that they needed to be controlled. Further exploration revealed that she would feel guilty and see herself as a bad person and that she did not like showing she was hurt.

> Ms. X: I think if he doesn't respond to me I'll get even more furious and upset. I'm thinking I would yell at him about ignoring me, but then I feel like a bad person.

Th: You must really struggle to manage these feelings, and I think in part it's because your mother couldn't tolerate them and made you feel bad for being upset at her.

Ms. X: I definitely feel that way. I don't like to show how I feel hurt either. I know I don't want to show that to you. I try not to cry in here.

Th: So I guess it's not just your anger but your hurt as well. I didn't know that you were purposely avoiding crying. We need to explore more about this, but I think it shows how much you have to guard against certain feelings. For the time being we don't really think that your husband would get so mad if you talked about his withdrawal, but I do think the longer you wait the more hurt and angry you get, making it even harder to say something.

Ms. X: That's true. It's very frustrating.

By the next session, after revealing her fears of showing hurt and vulnerability, the patient reported she was able to talk to her husband.

Th: So what happened?

Ms. X: It was kind of surprising. I told him how upset I was. He wasn't even aware of being distant. He didn't realize it was going on!

Th: So that's curious. He wasn't consciously rejecting you, if he was at all. Did you get any sense of what's going on with him?

Ms. X: You know, he really wasn't sure, but he did agree to go into therapy. He was very puzzled about it. And he became more engaged again.

Th: Okay. Well, that shows how important it is to continue to address this when it happens. I think we should get back to why you feel you need to be so in control with me.

In this case, the exploration of her difficulties discussing her hurt and frustration with her husband opened up the opportunity to explore new issues in the transference, as well as effect an important change in her behavior.

# Problems With Setting Limits With Children

Struggle with setting limits with children is a common behavioral difficulty, some examples of which have already been provided. In one pattern, parents can be overly lax about limit setting and then become increasingly frustrated about the child's abrogation of these limits. This can occur with younger children around such behaviors as scheduled bedtimes (typically efforts to delay them), time spent on computer games, or the number of products, such as toys or games, purchased. With adolescents behaviors such as curfews, social activities, and alcohol or drug use can become prominent. Children will often express anger around attempts to set limits, leading to power struggles between parents and children. Parents frequently become frustrated, possibly blaming the child for an inability to be satisfied or unwillingness to accept limits, often not recognizing their own role in the development of these fights. They may resort to a "crackdown" on limits, with consequences for noncompliance (e.g., withholding treasured activities from the child or grounding), leading to a temporary respite from problems. However, after a certain amount of time passes, these efforts tend to be relaxed, with an escalation of the preexisting pattern. Another problem that can occur is an overly rigid stance on the part of parents, not allowing children adequate opportunity to negotiate or challenge them.

Several factors can contribute to these limit-setting problems. Parents may believe that they were withheld from growing up, perhaps by overly strict parents, and that they want to be more giving to their children. Although potentially having a positive impact in avoiding rigidity, parents can overcompensate with a lack of proper limits. Another related contribution occurs when parents unconsciously equate setting limits with an identification with the aggressor, in which they fear that they are hurting their child; they frequently link such behavior with a parent they perceived as harsh and withholding. Parents may also wrestle with rageful feelings toward their children when challenges become severe, triggering guilt, defensive inhibitions, or overly severe expressions of anger. Although parents may indeed have harsh fantasies when frustrated, it is important to help them recognize that setting appropriate limits is actually a caring act toward a child, who needs to learn how to manage and tolerate frustration.

In addressing these problems, therapists can encourage setting firm but moderate limits, while exploring patients' inhibitions. The therapist can explain that when parents make clear that they will not budge on a limit, most children will give up their angry protest over time. They can communicate to children that with some behavior there is considerable freedom, with some there can be negotiation, and with other behavior there must be absolute boundaries (e.g., car seats or holding hands while crossing the street). However, many parents have trouble behaving differently after receiving such advice because these patterns are often deeply ingrained. Exploration of patients' fantasies and fears in limit setting is crucial in identifying ways to help them to behave in a more effective manner. As noted in the case below, many parents are not aware that they may give mixed messages about limits.

## Case Example

Ms. R (see Chapter 7) continued to struggle with setting limits with her children. At times she would be furious with her son, threatening to make him move out, and at other points go back to her more typical mode of taking care of him with little complaint, not addressing his failure to follow rules she had set in the house.

> Therapist: I think we've identified this pattern where you sometimes get furious with him and threaten to punish him or even kick him out, but at other points go back to business as usual. I don't think that you're aware of this pattern. However, it's important to recognize it, because otherwise it becomes difficult for you to set limits consistently. For instance, you want to have a set of rules that he needs to follow if he wants to live at home with you, such as keep his room clean, clean up the dishes, and not go out after midnight. But if you don't make that clear consistently he will probably assume he doesn't have to do it.
> Ms. R: Yeah. I didn't really realize that pattern. And I'm not really sure how to say those things to him. I don't want him to get mad.
> Th: Well, we can certainly discuss what your concerns are. But it's interesting that when you're upset you can be quite threatening to him and aren't worried about how he'll respond, but when you're calmer and can review rules with him you're frightened of getting him mad. I think it's important that we understand this, at the same time we discuss what you might say.
> Ms. R: I wonder why I might be like that.
> Th: We've talked how you were punished for being the most rebellious of the family, but we've also understood how you rebelled against what you saw as your parents' lack of involvement. I think you want to be more caring of your son than you felt. You don't want to be punitive like your parents were, but then you avoid maintaining any rules. Then every now and then your frustrations flare up and you become very critical.

Ms. R: I guess I can see what you're saying. I need to think about it. Do you know what I can do?
Th: I think you want to set clear limits and make sure not to backtrack from them. I think it would be good to be on the alert to when you feel like backtracking and to monitor what you are experiencing at that point. Then we can look at what you feel and consider how to address it.

Ms. R reduced her son's allowance, as he was not working, and he resisted looking for a job. However, at one point he asked if she would pay for him to join a gym.

Ms. R: So I said to him, "Well let's see how things are going with the job search," but then it turned out he hasn't been doing any searching.
Th: So what were you feeling after he asked?
Ms. R: Well, I found it kind of confusing. I was thinking that I should give the money because he should go to the gym. But I kind of doubt he would go anyway. He spends most of his day just hanging around with his friends. But I didn't want to get into a fight with him. Things had been going better. So I kind of waffled.
Th: Well, it sounds like you feel it would be harsh not to pay for the gym, but the problem is that it would be colluding with him if you did because it continues to send a message that he does not need to work. I think you could tell him that you need to stick with the rules because it's better for him to find a job and not be dependent on you.
Ms. R: Yes. I guess I didn't want to start a fight, but that's a good way of putting it. But overall he's actually fighting less since I've been clearer about limits.

Although some improvement occurred after these interventions, Ms. R continued to struggle intermittently with maintaining limits, even after she stated she would keep them in place. As she attempted to resist paying for more items for her son, she recognized another aspect of her difficulties.

Ms. R: So, I notice I'm wavering again about paying for the gym.
Th: What do you think is going on?
Ms. R: I'm not sure, but now he's bugging me about it. Not fighting.
Th: What does he say?

Ms. R: Well, he says, "Don't I think the gym would be good for him?" That way he could have more energy to do the things that he needs to do, like looking for a job.
Th: I know you've said that you think he's quite capable now of looking for work.
Ms. R: Yeah, but he guilts me into this.
Th: He may try to make you feel guilty, but you're the one hampered by guilt. What do you think you feel guilty about?
Ms. R: I feel like I'm just withholding something from him on principle that he could really use.
Th: It seems like you changed your mind about paying for the gym since we talked last. I wonder if guilt has been affecting you more than you thought. Maybe you feel like you are withholding from him just as your parents were inattentive to your needs.
Ms. R: That could be.
Th: It's important to remember that it's a very different circumstance. Your parents were distracted by their own interests and the conflicts between them. You are trying to set limits and help him be responsible.
Ms. R: So what could I say if I already waffled on it?
Th: I think you could say that you thought about it and you realized what's most important is helping him to be responsible to take care of things on his own. That it's really better for both of you. He can look for a job and then he will be able to pay for the gym himself.
Ms. R: I'll think about saying that.

## Case Example

As his therapy progressed, Mr. E (Chapters 3, 6, and 8) became aware that difficulties setting limits with his children involved internal conflicts that were related to those that inhibited his work efforts. The therapist and patient were able to clearly identify the point at which he struggled to impose consequences for his children's behavior, related to his guilt and fears of being a harsh and withholding parent.

Mr. E: I have done better with limit setting about their attitude and what they say to me. When they start saying hostile things, I tell them that it's unacceptable and has to stop. But when it comes to taking away things to get my son to do his homework, I'm having a hard time with it.
Th: We can look at why you've become more comfortable setting certain limits but not this one. What occurs to you as you do it?

Mr. E: I feel badly taking things away from him.

Th: But when you threaten to take the phone away and you don't take it, then it adds to a power struggle. You inadvertently enhance the pattern you're trying to prevent. Many parents are prone to that kind of pattern. It's important to understand why you have trouble being more consistent in the consequences you are using.

Mr. E: I feel guilty taking away his phone. It's important for him to keep in touch with friends.

Th: Well, you can talk with his therapist about other possible consequences. And we know you felt very deprived as a child, particularly after you had to move. But it's important to realize that setting a limit is actually a positive thing to do. It not only reduces power struggles but helps him learn to tolerate frustration.

Mr. E: Yes, I've been trying to tell myself that more.

Th: We need to see how we can help you to consider this at the time you're taking away the phone.

### Problems Identified by Others

Although some patients describe clear difficulties that they are contending with in their behavior, others present at the behest of family members or friends who have told them they have problems that are upsetting others. Many of these patients are reluctant to accept responsibility for these difficulties. These behaviors are not recognized as problematic or causing distress, as they are accepted as part of the personality or self. In such cases, the therapist helps patients to identify these behaviors as problematic and understand what contributes to them. The therapist not only works to identify strategies for intervening but also helps patients to recognize that these behaviors cause more distress for themselves and others than they realize.

#### Case Example

Mr. Y, a 62-year-old physical therapist, presented at the behest of his wife, reporting that he would voice criticism directly to others, often in a public setting, in a way that was upsetting for his wife and sometimes friends or relatives.

Therapist: Do you see this as being a problem?

Mr. Y: Well, my criticisms are on target. I don't think anyone would disagree with what I'm saying. But I guess she thinks I'm too blunt.

*Engaging the Patient in Addressing Specific Behavioral Problems* 133

> Th: Can you tell me about what happens?
> Mr. Y: There was an incident with her nephew that she says was the straw that broke the camel's back. It really bothered me what he was saying at a Christmas dinner. I'm annoyed about people who talk like they're so great when I know that actually they didn't do anything to get to the position that they're in.
> Th: What do you mean?
> Mr. Y: Well, he acts like he knows these important people through his work, and he's so important, but I know it was his Dad that got him the job. I just start getting furious. I let him have it. I told him he was full of himself and hadn't really accomplished anything on his own.
> Th: So I see that gets you furious. But I notice that not only does your behavior trouble your wife, but it also is upsetting for you in that you get really frustrated. Do you know why it bothers you so much?

Here the therapist reflects to the patient that his behavior and the associated feelings are troubling to himself as well as others. This strategy helps patients to recognize that expressing negative emotions, such as in the form of temper outbursts, can be an indication of underlying distress. In addition, patients suffer from the adverse impact on their relationships with others.

> Mr. Y: I haven't really thought about that. Maybe because I grew up in very tough circumstances. I wasn't given anything. And I wouldn't brag about overcoming that.
> Th: That makes sense. We should talk more about that.

As discussed in Chapter 5, "A Framework for Targeting Behavioral Change," monitoring what the patient experiences before behavior is useful in understanding what contributes to it and identifying points of intervention.

> Th: Is there anything that's been helpful at keeping these attacks from occurring?
> Mr. Y: I can try biting my tongue. Sometimes I just keep quiet, but it's difficult.
> Th: I think it would be good to see if you can try to hold back from being critical. That will make it easier to observe what you are experiencing at the time. And hopefully we can help

you to tolerate your feelings better when we understand more about them.

At the next visit Mr. Y reported an incident that had occurred in the interim.

Mr. Y: Well, I've been really good. No outbursts. But it wasn't easy. I have a couple of incidents I kept track of.
Th: That's encouraging, but it sounds like a struggle. What happened?
Mr. Y: Well, it's a friend of my wife's brother. He was showing off. I wanted to let him have it.
Th: What was he saying?
Mr. Y: It's hard to recall specifics.
Th: Are there any details you recall?
Mr. Y: Well, okay. He was going on and on about trips he was taking. He wanted to show off how much money he had. I happened to know he inherited a lot of his money. So what's the big deal? I think he's a phony.
Th: And that upsets you so much because…
Mr. Y: Nothing like that happened to me. I grew up in difficult times. My father was a tough guy. He worked hard all the time.
Th: Was he tough on you?
Mr. Y: Yeah, he was. I mean we weren't allowed to complain about anything. He would see that as weak. And it was a tough time. For many years we barely had enough to get by. I'm glad I've done better than that. But you won't hear me bragging about it.
Th: So perhaps that's part of why it bothers you so much. You had to struggle through these times. You're mad when others had it easier and they're bragging about it. But perhaps when they're bragging they're showing they're insecure about what they've accomplished.

The therapist's comment above is an example of the use of mentalizing to help modify patients' perspectives and feelings.

Mr. Y: I hadn't thought they might be insecure. It was rough growing up with my dad. He had a temper, even though we were good kids. I guess he was on edge. It felt like we bothered him a lot.

Th: So that affected you too I'm sure. Sounds like you couldn't complain, and didn't have much opportunity to express your anger.

Mr. Y: Oh, no. I guess I did get mad sometimes about his temper, but I wasn't going to say anything.

Th: So you must have really had difficulties when you felt angry.

Mr. Y: Yeah. And I notice it's hard for me even now. My anger really starts to build when I'm hearing people brag. I try to keep quiet, but then I kind of blow up and it comes out in an intense and mean way.

Th: I think these feelings from your background contribute to your anger. Understanding how you were affected by these experiences can help you to manage it better.

Mr. Y: I'll try thinking about these things when it happens next. I don't really want trouble with my wife and I don't want to be so bothered about these things!

## Impulse-Control Problems

Problems controlling impulses can occur in a variety of forms, such as temperamental outbursts of the type suffered by Mr. Y, struggles with expression of sexual wishes, and various forms of addictive behavior. These problems may be brought to the patient's attention by others, as in Mr. Y's case, or patients may experience painful feelings, such as guilt, in the context of having expressed impulses. For example, patients may regret enacting sexual behaviors with someone unlikely to be a long-term partner or outside their primary relationship. Or they may buy items when in debt or use drugs or alcohol, and then experience a plummet in self-esteem. More severe forms of these impulse disorders can require specialized treatment interventions, such as addiction specialists or rehab in the case of substance abuse. Psychodynamic psychotherapeutic approaches targeting behavior, however, can often be of value in modulating these difficult to control impulses, especially in less severe forms. As in the case below, identifying the context, feelings, and fantasies along with contributory dynamics can provide additional tools in regulating these behaviors.

### Case Example

Ms. Z, a 42-year-old sales representative, reported problems with managing her urges to buy expensive clothes and dinners, as well as gifts for her daughters. She rarely kept track of her expenses and would become frustrated when her husband complained about the size of their credit card bills. However, at other points she would realize the adverse impact on the family budget and become anxious and self-critical. The therapist worked with the patient to more consistently recognize the problematic nature of her spending urges and to become more aware of feelings and circumstances that might be triggers of her actions. At first very little information was obtained in this way, as Ms. Z would make these purchases reflexively and impulsively with limited awareness that it was occurring. The therapist also began to explore the patient's background and dynamics for clues to this problem.

Ms. Z characterized her early years as relatively normal, but starting about age 8 her parents began fighting more intensely and frequently. At age 10 her mother moved out of the family home, taking her clothes and some of the furniture with her, leaving her and her younger brother living with her father. The patient was only dimly aware, although she became increasingly so, that much of the family funds came from her mother's parents and that money was no longer available. Although her relationships with her father and brother were generally positive, they were all frustrated by a significant reduction in lifestyle and the need to move to a smaller house in a new area. In addition, her contacts with her mother were fairly limited, and she received little explanation from either parent about what happened in their relationship and how that affected her financially. She saw her mother more frequently as an adult, but had persistent anger at the level of separation and the reduction in finances that occurred at the time of the divorce, and viewed her mother as self-centered, with a focus on her own appearance. It also emerged over time that her mother had a drinking problem.

The therapist surmised that the patient's painful feelings around deprivation and abandonment, developing in part from the traumatic events at age 10, contributed to her buying urges. After he suggested these dynamics to the patient she became more aware of the context of her spending.

> Ms. Z: So I have noticed that I go shopping or make these reservations at fancy restaurants right after I feel frustrated with something that's happened to me or angry at someone.
> Therapist: Can you give me some specific instances?
> Ms. Z: Well, the other day I got furious with my husband. He's been working harder, but not really making any more money. He says he's going to be home at a certain time, but then he'll get home an hour or two after that. I'm worn out taking care of the boys and I get very frustrated. I feel I have to handle everything by myself.

Th: That comment is interesting, because it sounds like how you may have felt when your mother left—abandoned and deprived—and feeling you had to manage more on your own.

Ms. Z: I didn't realize that, but I see the connection. That's interesting because the other instance I was going to tell you about was after I got mad at her.

Th: What happened then?

Ms. Z: I called her up to talk to her about a problem with my friend. I'm not sure if maybe she was drinking, but she didn't seem to be paying any attention to what I was saying. I said, "You're not even listening to me," and she said, "I can't talk right now," and got off the phone. I was furious and just headed out shopping. I did feel better after buying some things.

Th: So this pattern suggests that you're wrestling with feeling abandoned and deprived, as well as angry. The shopping appears to be a way to shut down or ease those feelings. But the problem is that it creates difficulties for you both in terms of managing your finances and gaining a better understanding of what's going on inside. If you're mad at your husband or feel abandoned, we want you to have a way to address this rather than shop.

Ms. Z: Well, abandonment does kind of capture how I felt at age 10, and later I did feel deprived. I used to get a lot of stuff before my Mom moved out and then that just ended suddenly. But I'll have to see what I can do because I really don't think of these things before I shop.

Th: I think you're already more attuned to what's going on inside before you head out to a store. The more you pay attention and the better you understand what triggers your behaviors, the greater the opportunity to stop yourself. It's like constructing a scaffolding around a building to help step back from it. You can better identify what's wrong and be in a better position to fix it.

This metaphor was referred to in Chapter 5 as a way to help patients understand how they might intervene in their own problematic behaviors.

Ms. Z: Okay, I'll keep trying to pay more attention. Now sometimes I think before I do it. Other times I don't.

In a subsequent session Ms. Z informed the therapist about progress in this effort.

Ms. Z: You're right about my feeling deprived and mad before I buy things. I don't really think of my Mom at that point, but I am thinking about how someone's causing me trouble: either my husband not helping me, or my kids being demanding, or my boss putting pressure on me to make more sales. The urge to buy is really strong, but a couple times I have been able to stop it.

Th: How do you feel when you do this?

Ms. Z: I do feel good about it, but my feelings of frustration are pretty strong. Sometimes I'll start yelling at the family, and I don't like to do this. It reminds me of my Mom.

Th: I think it's important to understand that link to your Mom at that point, but I also think it's an opportunity to learn new ways to manage your frustration.

Ms. Z: Okay. Well, we better start working on those.

Over the course of several sessions the patient continued to focus on the origins of her anger and how it might be better managed. One problem she had was limit setting with her children, as discussed above. The therapist and patient identified that she did not want her children to be deprived, as she had felt. However, her constant willingness to buy them new toys or clothes led them to expect these items whenever they were frustrated. Ms. Z, initially unaware of this pattern, would become angry about their demands.

Th: I understand your wish that your children not be too deprived, but I think you overcompensate for your own feelings when you are always buying things for them. That can make it hard for them to manage their own frustrations, and it certainly gets you upset when they keep asking you for things.

Ms. Z: You mean I'm causing them to be this way?

Helping patients to identify their own behaviors as the source of certain problems can sometimes lead to their having negative reactions, including denial, anger, or guilt. They can perceive the therapist as judging or blaming them. Sometimes it can be useful to examine these reactions in the context of the transference, whereas in other instances it may be appropriate to reassure patients that they are not doing these things intentionally, and understanding them better can help them to reverse a pattern that can lead to further problems over time.

> Th: I don't think you're doing it intentionally. But I think it has to do with some of the same issues you have. You certainly would not want them to experience what you did. But making changes can help your children to learn to deal better with their own frustrations and help you to be less annoyed with them.
> Ms. Z: Well, that's interesting. I had no idea these same problems might be affecting them. But what do I do when they're so demanding?
> Th: It might be useful to let them know that you're not going to be buying them things as frequently now because you don't think it's good for them, but I think we're going to need to help you tolerate your feelings and their frustration when you make these changes.
> Ms. Z: Yes, because it's similar to the shopping for myself. I just forget and start buying stuff.

Another factor that emerged over time was the idea that these items symbolized a more consistently present mother, or the return of her mother to her life when she was an adolescent. However, she was recurrently disappointed, as these products could not possibly be a replacement for her mother. In this way Ms. Z needed to further mourn the loss of a wished-for mother who was more responsive or empathic.

> Ms. Z: Now every time I'm about to buy something, I stop and ask myself why do I need this? Why am I feeling deprived? And I notice things don't mean as much to me as they used to.
> Th: For a lot of people, things mean some kind of love or caring or feeding, but they end up dissatisfied because these items don't really equate to what another person can offer.
> Ms. Z: Yes. I know you've said that before, and I'm getting a better idea of what you mean. So I guess these things have become less important as I've recognized this. But I still like to shop, believe me. I just feel I have more control than I used to. I miss it.

# Addressing Behavioral Problems Related to Adverse Developmental Experiences and Trauma

Many sources of evidence point to the role of adverse developmental experiences and trauma in the development of a broad range of symptoms and problematic behavior (Casey and Strain 2016; Kessler et al. 2010). Although obtaining the history in the initial consultation will elicit some episodes of trauma, patients may not reveal other incidents because they are ashamed, do not connect the trauma to their current symptoms, or may have repressed the event(s). Sometimes patients (and therapists) avoid exploring traumatic and painful childhood experiences because of the emotional distress they trigger. Therefore, clinicians should be alert to the potential emergence of further information about trauma in the course of treatment. In addition, in the context of persistent posttraumatic symptoms such as phobias, affective dysregulation, and dissociation, therapists should consider additional exploration of traumatic events. This investigation will often identify sources and dynamics, along with points of intervention, for recurrently problematic behaviors. Many of the patients in the examples thus far in this book had histories of trauma and/or adverse developmental experiences that were relevant to their treatment, and this chapter focuses in depth on addressing the impact of these experiences on behavior. Although this chapter focuses on psychodynamic approaches to posttraumatic symptoms, a broad range of interventions may be necessary for effective treatment of these problems (Casey and Strain 2016).

The impact of traumatic events can be wide ranging (Busch et al. 2012; Kessler et al. 2010; Silove et al. 2015). Adverse developmental experiences, particularly with caregivers, can create an insecure attachment style, which increases vulnerability to subsequent traumatic and harmful events. Potential consequences include disruptions in the sense of self, flashbacks of the trauma, dissociative experiences, anxiety and/or irritability, and a range of problematic behaviors. Patients may unconsciously repeat the trauma, either viewing dissimilar events as being like the trauma or inadvertently engaging in or provoking experiences reminiscent of the trauma. Intrapsychic conflicts surrounding aggression and separation are heightened by traumatic events, along with intensification of negative emotions (including rage and fear) and polarized self/other representations (e.g., victim and victimizer). Longings for intimacy may be threatening because of feelings of vulnerability and mistrust.

Defensive reactions include dissociation, in which numbness or a disconnect of memories and emotions attempt to blunt intensely painful feelings; repression, in which fantasies and memories that create pain and anxiety are kept from conscious awareness; identification with the aggressor; and counterphobic behavior, in which patients may enact behavior that aims to deny the impact of traumatic events. Guilt and shame may be prominent, with an intense or persistent self-blame for traumatic events and a felt need for punishment. Traumatic sequelae also frequently include somatic symptoms, which may represent traumatic experiences that have not symbolized, symbolic expressions of conflicts, or a defense against intrapsychic conflicts or painful memories (Busch 2017).

In this chapter we will consider behavioral problems stemming from trauma and adverse childhood experiences (Table 11–1), including unconscious repetition, difficulties associated with identification with the aggressor, phobic symptoms, problematic parental behavior, expressions of irritability, and somatic preoccupations.

**TABLE 11–1.** Behavioral problems related to trauma

Repetition of traumatic experiences
Identification with the aggressor
Problematic parental behavior in response to trauma
Phobic behavior
Expressions of irritability
Somatic preoccupations

## Repetition of Traumatic Experiences

Freud (1920/1955) described how patients inadvertently tend to repeat traumatic episodes, either intrapsychically or in their behavior or relationship with others, referring to this phenomenon as "repetition compulsion" (Corradi 2009). For example, individuals who have been abused in childhood may inadvertently become involved in relationships with problematic partners that heighten the potential for a recurrence of being abused. Several factors can contribute to such behavior, such as an unconscious wish to master or control the trauma in which the patient felt helpless, a wish to punish others for abuse the patient experienced, or a sense that abuse is necessary for intense closeness to occur. A background of trauma is often relevant to various forms of unexplained self-destructive behavior, such as drug abuse, self-injury, and suicidal behavior, which can represent, in part, a form of self-induced reexperiencing of the trauma.

### Case Example

Ms. F (see Chapters 3, 6, 7, and 9), who described a history of adverse parental reactions to a broad array of her needs, moved forward with a plan for renovations of her home. After an agreement was made with an architect and contractor, the architect began to tell Ms. F that her plans were unworkable and that he needed to proceed with a new design for the renovation. Ms. F was very upset when this occurred as she was happy with the current plan. She wanted to tell the architect to stop pressing her and that she wanted to proceed without changes. However, as in instances with her son and others, she was fearful of expressing her feelings, and also began to question her own judgment.

> Therapist: What are you worried will happen if you tell him that you want to proceed as you did originally?

Ms. F: I'm worried he'll get furious with me and maybe even quit. I actually did question his ideas a bit after we talked the other day and he did get mad. He raised his voice a bit and said it wasn't going to work the way I want it.

Th: This sounds like you're frightened just like you were with your mother. That it's not safe to express your own opinion. It's like you're caught in a repeat of the traumatic experiences you had with her.

Ms. F: I hear what you're saying. And I do feel frozen. I feel I'm stuck in a terrible position.

Th: I think it's important to consider how different this situation is from that with your mother, even though it feels similar. First, it's not very professional for him to get angry and threaten to quit when he originally agreed to your plans. And what if he quits? Maybe he's not right to do the job if you disagree with how he's doing it.

M. F: Well, I guess that all sounds rational. I didn't realize how much it felt like my mother. But I'm scared to say these things.

Th: I think we need to consider that you're vulnerable to repeating these kinds of situations based on the experiences you've had. I guess one other idea is to have your husband talk to him.

Ms. F: Well I've thought about doing that. I actually have talked to Bill and he's worried about how I'm stuck. He doesn't like to get involved with these things, but maybe he'd consider it.

## Identification With the Aggressor

Identification with the aggressor is another important element to be alert to in assessing the impact of trauma on behavior. In employing this defense, patients may identify with the perpetrator of the trauma or others who have had power and control over them. Such an identification may be experienced in fantasy or enacted with others, for example, bullying others as one has been bullied. Fantasies or wishes to harm others as one has been harmed can create significant guilt and distress, adding greatly to inhibitions in behavior. For example, a mother who has been physically abused as a child can struggle with fears/wishes related to harming her own child, leading to inadequate limit setting. In the example below, Mr. T, discussed in Chapter 9 ("Working With Sustaining Behavioral Change and the Response of Others"), who had been bullied by his father, wrestled with wishes and fears around controlling his own children.

## Case Example

Mr. T became enraged at his children when they did not do what he expected. In an example of dissociative tendencies caused by trauma, he was furious at his own father's controlling behavior and had vowed not to reenact it with his children, even as he felt the urge to compel them to yield to his authority. The therapist's pointing out to Mr. T how Mr. T's father's attitudes infiltrated his thoughts and feelings aided him in reevaluating his approach to his children.

> Mr. T: I told you that my children are not respectful of me. They don't want to participate in any of the plans that I set up for them.
> Therapist: Well, I don't think that's unusual for teenagers. What was your plan?
> Mr. T: I wanted to take them to a movie. But they just complained about going. They don't show me any respect.
> Th: I'm not really sure this is about respect for you. I don't think they want to be caught in the trap.

"Caught in the trap" was Mr. T's shorthand way of describing the complex feelings he had with his authoritarian father, with Mr. T believing that he had no say in what he wanted to do in his life and that his father was domineering.

> Mr. T: So you don't think I should tell them they have to go to the movie?
> Th: Well, I recognize that in some instances you would have to be firm with them, but I'm not sure about this one. You yourself said that you don't want to put them in a trap like your father did with you. I think sometimes you don't recognize how your father's attitudes or behavior might emerge in you. You might be identifying with him without realizing it.
> Mr. T: Yes, I do recognize that I might bully others in some circumstances. And I don't want to do that with the kids, but I also think I'm afraid to take a firmer stance, because I want everyone to like me.

This statement was a shorthand for another impact from his father's bullying and critical behavior. Feeling pressured by his father, he had become aware of needing to please others, for fear of getting rejected or punished. This tendency interfered with his capacity to set appropriate limits with his children and others. Patients may at times fear asserting themselves with others and in other situations be demanding and bullying. This type of split is not unusual as a consequence of developmental trauma; individuals often do not recognize that they are experiencing or behaving in these contradictory ways. The therapist works to help patients integrate these conflicting aspects. In Mr. T's case, the therapist explored how he was being affected by the trauma, and worked on integrating the split-off aspects and enabling a gradient of response to his children's behavior.

> Th: I think you're talking about two very different reactions to your father's behavior that make it hard for you in reacting to your children. On the one hand you may identify with him in trying to make them do a specific activity, and on the other hand be fearful of setting necessary limits because you feel you need to please them. I think understanding the different ways you are affected would make it easier for you to figure out where to draw the line.
> Mr. T: Well, that makes sense. Thinking about it that way, I'm not sure why I was so insistent on the movie. But I'm not sure what to do when they visit then.
> Th: You could ask them more about what they want to do.
> Mr. T: I think they'll want to just sit home and work on their computers, but I'll ask.

## Problematic Parental Behavior in Response to Trauma

One area of the impact of trauma is on the experience and behavior of parents in relation to children. Clinical observations and research indicate how a child may behave in ways that trigger recollection of past traumatic experiences, resulting in negative reactions on the part of the parent. This behavior can lead to reflexive reactions that can become instantiated in problematic interactional patterns. For instance, normal inconsolability in a child can remind an individual of a mother who was either unresponsive to her needs or demanding of an excessive amount of comforting or "parenting" on the part of the child. The patient might respond with angry withdrawal, blaming ("Why are you doing this to me?"), or excessive responsiveness to the child's tension, rather than a measured effort to help the child process the negative emotions and reactions. These problematic patterns of interaction can benefit from elucidating the link of the traumatic experiences to adverse behavior.

### Case Example

Ms. Q (see Chapters 6 and 7) complained about her daughter's unwillingness or irritable reactions when the patient would request a visit. However, she had trouble considering that her daughter might have been trying to set boundaries in terms of time spent with her. "She doesn't care about me. Maybe it's because of how she felt I treated her father," Ms. Q would aver, despite it being evident that her daughter was quite involved with her. Exploration brought to mind her own relationship with her mother, in which she experienced herself as the parent attempting to soothe her mother's catastrophic preoccupations. Ms. Q believed there was a lack of boundaries and felt guilty about her own attempts to set limits with her mother. She had been careful to not pressure her daughter to respond to her needs and worries as her mother would with her, but then felt frustrated that her daughter was not more responsive. Also, Ms. Q was indirectly expressing anger she felt toward her mother, who ultimately was unresponsive to the patient's needs. In addition, she felt the urge to coerce her daughter to respond, a form of identification with the aggressor, which then caused her to have a wave of guilty feelings. This guilt and concerns about her anger contributed to difficulties addressing these problems directly. After these dynamics and possible behavioral scripts were addressed, Ms. Q was able to have a breakthrough with her daughter:

> Ms. Q: I told her that she and I were stuck in this pattern and I wanted to try to find a way out of it. I accepted part of the blame and that I would get frustrated about the limits she set.
> Therapist: So how did that go?
> Ms. Q: She was much more responsive than I expected. It went very well after that. I talked some about my medical problems and she seemed willing to listen. I'm worried about whether it will continue.
> Th: Well, I think we need to continue to examine the times when you get frustrated with her and we can recall how you handled it differently.
> Ms. Q: Also, you can remind me about how much I'm still affected by my mother. I didn't realize that those problems I had with her still affected me so much.
> Th: Yes, I agree we need to continue to sort through the anger and guilt you had about her.

# Phobic Behavior

Although multiple factors can contribute, phobic symptoms and behavior at the level of a disorder are a common outcome of trauma (Busch et al. 2012). Many individuals with more severe forms of such avoidance grew up in environments that were frightening or neglectful. To a degree, such phobic behavior can be viewed as adaptive learning that is displaced to the world at large (assuming the individual's current environment is relatively safe) or specific types of experiences (e.g., flying, public bathrooms). A learning model is useful in understanding and addressing some aspects of avoidance, but psychodynamic approaches can be used to identify underlying dynamics and meanings of symptoms and behaviors to understand posttraumatic reactions and develop points of intervention. The therapist is interested in how the traumatic experiences have become internalized in the form of fantasy, intrapsychic conflict, defense, symptom, and avoidant behavior.

An initial step of this approach is to identify the probable connections between the phobic behavior and the traumatic event. In many instances an individual does not recognize the relationship because the link has never been suggested and/or dissociative tendencies or defenses have blocked the conscious experience of the connection between the experience and painful feelings that are triggered. Identifying the link is an important step in developing a framework for addressing the behavior, such as with the comment, "I wonder if you are so frightened of people in authority because of the harsh punishments you frequently received from your father." In addition to noting the connection to trauma, this genetic interpretation also suggests that the patient is overly fearful of authority in the current circumstances. In an example of going beyond a model of learned expectations, the therapist might comment, if appropriate, on the patient's struggle with angry feelings and fantasies toward authority that contribute to avoidance, because the intensity of these emotions can be frightening, creating intrapsychic conflict.

After such links and dynamics are identified, the therapist can work with the patient in clarifying that the phobic dangers are not realistic or at all likely in the present situation, but instead are derived from past traumatic experiences and internal fears. The therapist can then employ the varying behavioral interventions elaborated in the prior chapters of this book. Phobic behaviors can take many forms beyond the usual fears of specific situations. The most common phobic symptom discussed in these chapters is the fear of directly confronting others and self-assertion, many instances of which have been described. Mr. T, for example, was phobic about asserting himself at work, concerned that his colleagues and boss would be competitive and retaliatory. Understanding how these fears were linked to painful developmental experiences helped him to more assertively seek and obtain new clients. Confirmation of the difference between his current situation and childhood circumstances came as the feared backlash did not occur.

## Expressions of Irritability

Posttraumatic symptoms often include anxiety and irritability, sometimes alternating with dissociative states. As with other symptoms, patients frequently do not connect angry feelings and behaviors to traumatic and other adverse experiences. Patients often have underlying rage at perpetrators of the trauma, or others they believe did not protect them. These feelings are frequently displaced toward intimate partners or authority figures not involved in these events. Complicating these circumstances, patients may alternate between inhibitions of assertiveness in some situations and over-aggressiveness in others, each potentially linked to the traumatic experiences. Identifying this variability, connecting the symptoms to the trauma, and identifying behavioral alternatives can aid patients in managing their expression of these feelings toward others.

### Case Example

Mr. AA was a 46-year-old corporate lawyer who developed PTSD following the loss of coworkers on 9/11. He initially avoided severe symptoms through taking the role of a "super worker" at the office, working overtime to keep the firm functioning. However, after several months he became disillusioned with this endeavor, particularly since the firm made little effort to address the emotional impact of the loss of colleagues. He became increasingly anxious and depressed and felt either disconnected from or irritable with his wife. He presented for psychiatric treatment, and his symptoms showed a partial response to sertraline. The therapist identified that the recent trauma confirmed long-standing feelings of mistrust and aloneness. In exploring Mr. AA's early life, the patient described how he felt a need to be the "good boy" for his mother to support her dealings with an abusive, alcoholic father. The efforts reminded him of his "super worker" role at his company, as there was also little acknowledgment in the family of his anger and guilt at both parents regarding their behavior.

As Mr. AA worked through these feelings in psychotherapy, his symptoms improved further, but he began to manifest recurrent conflicts with authority figures. For instance, he argued with his boss about being overworked and fought with his landlord about what he believed was poor management of his apartment. In response, his boss reprimanded him and his landlord threatened to not extend his lease. Although in part these actions represented an advance in gaining access to anger that was previously repressed or self-directed, he and the therapist were concerned that his aggressive stance was putting his job and apartment at risk. They focused on targeting these behaviors directly.

> Therapist: What happens when you feel like fighting with your boss?
>
> Mr. AA: I just think about how much work I'm getting and how I can't get home in the evening to relax, and he doesn't even care about it.
>
> Th: And then what happens when you confront him?
>
> Mr. AA: I tell him this is ridiculous. It's too much. And he keeps saying I have to do the work. And then I feel guilty and get really worried about the job.
>
> Th: Has he threatened your job?
>
> Mr. AA: No. Not yet anyway. But I think he may be getting fed up.
>
> Th: What do you feel guilty about?
>
> Mr. AA: I think: Now I'm making him feel bad. And I don't know if there's anything he can do about it. He's under pressure too.
>
> Th: This sounds like the pattern we've talked about. These authorities remind you of your father or perhaps those who perpetrated 9/11. You're furious at them for what they've done, but then you feel guilty and anxious. You worry you're a bully too, like them.
>
> Mr. AA: I see what you're saying. But then I also feel helpless, like I did when I was a kid. I thought I was improving by saying something.
>
> Th: Well, I think it's true that we've helped you to have more access to your anger and stand up for yourself. You have a right to feel furious, but I think you need to work more on how you tolerate and express these feelings. Your anger is stoked by your traumatic experiences and the way you express it to your boss seems to heighten the conflict with him and cause you to feel guilty and worried. Perhaps we can discuss what you might say to him that would be more helpful. Maybe you could sit down with him and talk about ways of managing the work load rather than getting enraged every now and then.

Mr. AA: I think that's a good point about how these traumas have fueled my anger. Maybe that's why it feels over the top with him. Maybe knowing that can help me handle the feelings better. They do kind of surge up.

Understanding these manifestations of his anger about the traumatic events helped him to modulate these impulses, as he became aware of the intensity of his rage toward those who had harmed him, and how much he wished to retaliate. The therapist and he determined that part of what continued to make him so anxious and angry was his unconscious wish to and fear of harming others, making him an abuser in his fantasy, another example of identification with the aggressor. As he found that this wish was understandable in the context of what he had experienced, he felt less threatened by and more in control of these urges.

## Somatic Preoccupations With Trauma

Somatic symptoms and catastrophic fears about them are common sequelae of trauma and can lead to problematic behaviors such as avoidance of work or preoccupations that adversely impact relationships. For example, Ms. I's husband's health care worries (see Chapters 4, 5, 7, and 8) affected his relationship with his wife and his employability. These symptoms can represent aspects of trauma that have not been translated into the symbolic, verbal sphere (Busch 2017). In addition, somatic preoccupations can function as a defense against painful or frightening intrapsychic conflicts; patients avoid conscious access to these experiences through a focus on the body. They can also symbolize an underlying intrapsychic conflict. Understanding the link to trauma and relevant dynamics can aid in diminishing these symptoms and associated behavioral difficulties.

### Case Example

Mr. BB, a 46-year-old advertising executive, presented with recurrent hypochondriacal fears and conflicts at work. He felt that he was mistreated by his boss, not getting proper credit for his contributions. By attending to context, the therapist and patient determined that his somatic symptoms would intensify when he believed that there was evidence of his being overlooked. Rather than confronting problems with his boss directly, however, Mr. BB would withdraw and become sullen. He described a background in which he was shuttled between his divorced parents and felt neglected in both of their homes. He described his mother as dysfunctional and struggling with drug problems. His father had a new wife with her own children, and he felt like a second-class citizen. He recalled feeling angry, rejected, and helpless; any efforts to complain about the situation went unheeded, or he was criticized for creating trouble. The therapist and patient were able to link his behavior and fears at work to his traumatic developmental experiences. As in his childhood home, he believed confronting problems with his boss to be too dangerous, yet his behavior was creating increased tension at work.

This new understanding helped him to consider trying to address his problems more directly. Therapist and patient discussed possible comments to make to his boss regarding the unfairness he was experiencing, including his belief that his compensation was inadequate. These discussions did not trigger the conflict he anticipated. In fact, he became less withdrawn and the boss became somewhat friendlier, and his somatic concerns eased considerably. However, the boss did not increase his salary.

He began to look at other possible employment opportunities and quickly found a job at another company. After the move to the new job, Mr. BB was very pleased but noticed a resurgence in hypochondriacal worries, particularly when he was alone on the weekend. He had trouble understanding this anxiety, as everything was going so well with the job and at home.

> Therapist: What comes to mind about being alone?
> Mr. BB: I hadn't considered this before, but I felt very alone on the weekends with my mom.
> Th: What would happen?
> Mr. BB: She would be busy with all kinds of things like social activities and part time work, and I was usually just left at home. If I had been with my father I could have gone out with friends, but I didn't know anyone where she lived.
> Th: How old were you then?
> Mr. BB: Six to twelve.
> Th: That's a young age to leave a kid at home alone.
> Mr. BB: Oh, yeah. It was lonely; and scary! And you know, my father didn't really care. No one seemed to be paying any attention to my needs.
> Th: Did you ever consider saying anything?
> Mr. BB: If I complained my father didn't seem interested because my stepmom needed me to be away. If I complained to my mother she would send me on a big guilt trip, saying how we had such little time together and that she was really hurt that I wanted to spend time with my dad or my friends and not her.
> Th: So you really felt trapped then.

Mr. BB: Yeah I did. Somehow now that I'm in this new situation, these fears are coming back to me.

The realization of aloneness in these new circumstances helped Mr. BB to understand the source of his resurgence in his somatic fears. These symptoms eased with this recognition and as he became closer to colleagues in his new environment. In the new work setting he felt more respected and worked to avoid the patterns of withdrawal that had occurred previously, making efforts to address problems more directly.

## References

Busch FN: A model for integrating actual neurotic or unrepresented states and symbolized aspects of intrapsychic conflict. Psychoanal Q 86(1):75–108, 2017 28272818

Busch FN, Milrod BL, Singer M, et al: Panic-Focused Psychodynamic Psychotherapy—eXtended Range. New York, Routledge, 2012

Casey PR, Strain JJ (eds): Trauma and Stressor-Related Disorders. Arlington, VA, American Psychiatric Press, 2016

Corradi RB: The repetition compulsion in psychodynamic psychotherapy. J Am Acad Psychoanal Dyn Psychiatry 37(3):477–500, 2009 19764847

Freud S: Beyond the pleasure principle (1920), in Standard Edition of the Complete Psychological Works of Sigmund Freud, Vol 18. Translated and edited by Strachey J. London, Hogarth Press, 1955, pp 1–64

Kessler RC, McLaughlin KA, Green JG, et al: Childhood adversities and adult psychopathology in the WHO World Mental Health Surveys. Br J Psychiatry 197(5):378–385, 2010 21037215

Silove D, Alonso J, Bromet E, et al: Pediatric-onset and adult-onset separation anxiety disorder across countries in the world mental health survey. Am J Psychiatry 172(7):647–656, 2015 26046337

# Index

Page numbers printed in **boldface** type refer to tables.

Abandonment, in case example, 136
Abstinence, and avoidance of focus on behavioral change in psychoanalysis, **2**, 3
Active therapy, 2
Adaptive learning, and phobic behavior, 148
Addictive behavior, and impulse-control problems, 135
Adverse reactions, of others to behavioral change, 120–122
Affects. *See also* Anger
    elaborating of feelings and fantasies about performance of alternative behaviors, 62
    framework for examining context, affects, and meanings of problematic behavior, 60, **74**
    identifying circumstances, affects, and meanings surrounding problematic behaviors, 76–79
    intrapsychic conflicts and negative affects from behavioral change, 112–113
Aggression. *See* Identification with aggressor
Agoraphobia, 33
Alternative behaviors. *See also* Behavioral change; Problematic behaviors
    collaborative approach to, 88–92
    framework for targeting of behavioral change and, **56**, 61, 62
    homework and, 108–110
    identification of specific factors interfering with, 102–108
    scripts for, 87, **88**, 92–99
    techniques for identification of, **88**
Anger
    defense mechanisms and, 46–47
    determining problematic behavior and, 56
    expression of in power struggles between parents and children, 128
    identifying context, fantasies, and emotions triggering, 79–81, 83
    scripts for alternative behaviors and, 97
    working through and, 53
Anxiety. *See also* Generalized anxiety disorder; Separation anxiety
    in case examples, 34, 58, 91, 116

Anxiety (*continued*)
　　as interfering factors in implementation of alternative behaviors, 102
Assertiveness
　　in case example, 17–23
　　defense mechanisms and, **14**, 15–16, 49
　　in determining whether behavior is problematic, 56–57
　　impact of developmental factors and traumatic experiences on, 14–15
　　intrapsychic conflicts and, **14**, 15
　　mentalization and, **14**, 16–17, 18, 20, 22, 23
　　personality difficulties and, **14**, 16
　　psychodynamic factors inhibiting, **14**
　　struggles with in implementation of alternative behaviors, 102–105
　　working definition of, 13
　　working through and, 53
Attachment, and problematic behaviors related to development experiences, 23, 53, 142
Attack and counterattack patterns, and couples therapy, 124
Avoidance
　　as defense in case example, 117
　　phobic behavior as outcome of trauma and, 148
　　of scripts, 94

Behavioral change. *See also* Alternative behaviors; Problematic behaviors; Psychodynamic approaches
　　changing views on interventions for in psychoanalysis, 4–6
　　dealing with forms of that do not generalize, 113–116
　　framework for targeting of, 55, **56,** 57–71
　　intrapsychic conflicts and negative affects from, 112–113
　　potential problems in targeting of, vii, 1–4, 27, **28,** 29–40
　　psychoanalytic techniques for addressing, 6–11, 41, **42**
　　psychodynamic understanding of factors impeding, 13–24
　　response of others to, 117–122
　　working with as aid to psychoanalytic goals, 10, **11**
　　working with degree and impact of, **113**
Behavior therapy, integration of psychoanalysis and, 8. *See also* Cognitive-behavioral therapy
Borderline personality disorder, and reflective functioning, 16
Bullying
　　in case example, 120–121
　　identification with aggressor as defense mechanism and, 144, 145, 146

Case examples
　　of collaborative approach, 39–40, 88–90, 91–92
　　of countertransference, 37–38
　　of defense mechanisms, 47, 48–50
　　of dependency of patient on therapist, 29–32
　　of development of mentalization skills, 52–53
　　of framework for targeting behavioral change, 57, 58, 59, 62–67, 70–71

of generalization of behavioral change, 114–116
of homework for implementing alternative behaviors, 109–110
of identification with aggressor as response to trauma, 145
of identifying factors interfering with alternative behaviors, 103–106, 107–108
of identifying triggers of angry behavior, 80
of impulse-control problems, 135–139
of interpretation of problematic behavior, 44–46
of intrapsychic conflicts and negative affects from behavioral change, 112–113
of irritability as posttraumatic symptom, 149–151
of marital and couples' problems, 124–127
of multiple contributors to problematic behavior, 84–85
of pragmatic psychodynamic psychotherapy, 5–6
of problematic parental behavior in response to trauma, 147
of problems identified by others, 132–135
of procrastination in behavioral change, 77–79
of psychodynamic formulation, 17–23, 81–82, 83
of repetition of traumatic experiences, 143–144
of response of others to behavioral change, 118–122
of scripts for alternative behaviors, 93–99
of self-observational capacity, 75–76
of setting of limits with children, 129–132
of somatic preoccupations with trauma, 151–153
of therapeutic relationship, 29–32, 33, 34–35
of unassertiveness, 17–23
Children. *See also* Developmental factors; Parenting
abuse of and identification with aggressor in, 144
abuse of and repetition of traumatic experiences, 143
problems with setting limits for, 127–132, 138
Clarification, as technique for addressing behavioral change, 42–43, 44
Cognitive-behavioral therapy. *See also* Behavior therapy
development of approaches to behavioral change in, vii–viii
homework and, 68
symptom substitution and, 3
therapeutic relationship in, 28–29
Collaborative approach, to psychodynamic psychotherapy for behavioral change, **29,** 38–40, 88–92
Conflict, and interpretation as technique for addressing behavioral change, **42,** 44, 45. *See also* Intrapsychic conflicts
Confrontation, as technique for addressing behavioral change, 42–43
Context, and meanings of problematic behavior, 60, **74,** 79–81

Counterphobic behavior, and traumatic sequelae, 142
Countertransference
  in case example, 121
  potential problems in targeting of behavioral change and, **28, 29,** 36–38
  use of as technique for addressing behavioral change, 53–54
Couples therapy
  marital problems and, 123–127
  scripts and, 95–96

Defense mechanisms. *See also* Dissociation; Identification with aggressor; Incompetence; Passive aggression; Reaction formation
  humor as, 98
  interpretation of as technique for addressing behavioral change, **42,** 44, 46–51
  psychodynamic formulation of factors contributing to problematic behavior and, 60–61
  traumatic sequelae and, 142
  unassertiveness as factor contributing to behavior problems and, **14,** 15–16
Dependency
  in case example, 48–49
  potential adverse impact of patient's on therapist in therapeutic relationship, 28–32
Depression, in case examples, 29, 34, 91
Developmental factors. *See also* Children
  assertiveness and, 14–15
  in case examples, 18, 40, 66, 115
  identifying contributors to problematic behavior and, 76
  potential consequences of adverse experiences of, 142
  psychodynamic formulation of factors contributing to problematic behavior and, 60–61
Diary
  as form of homework, 69, 109
  monitoring of context, affects, and meanings of problematic behavior with, 74
Dissociation
  in case examples, 38, 94
  as defensive reaction to trauma, 142
Distress, and somatic symptoms in case example, 103
Dysthymia, in case example, 47

Enactments, and transference, 52
Escitalopram, in case example, 91
Experiential learning, and time-limited dynamic psychotherapy, 9

Family. *See* Children; Marriage; Parenting
Fantasies
  confrontation of specific in psychoanalytic process, 10
  identification with aggressor and, 144
  identifying context and emotions triggering angry behavior, 79–81
  inadequacy and, 105
  of patients about outcome of behavioral change, 120

performance of alternative
    behaviors and, 62
  of rescue in case example, 108
Fear
  confrontation of specific in
    psychoanalytic process, 10
  identification of behavioral
    alternatives and, 99
Ferenczi, S., 2
Free association, as technique for
  addressing behavioral change,
  41–42
Freud, Sigmund, vii, vii, 1–2, 112,
  143

Generalization, of behavioral change,
  113–116
Generalized anxiety disorder, in case
  example, 5
Genetic interpretation, as technique
  for addressing behavioral
  change, **42,** 44
Gratification, contrasted to technical
  stance of abstinence, 3
Guilt
  behavioral scripts and, 96
  in case example, 121–122
  as interfering factor in
    implementation of alternative
    behaviors, 102–103
  of patient about favorable life
    changes, 112
  traumatic sequelae and, 142

Homework
  framework for targeting
    behavioral change and, **56,**
    68–71
  identifying and addressing factors
    interfering with alternative
    behaviors and, **103**

time-limited dynamic
  psychotherapy and, 9
use of in implementing alternative
  behaviors, 108–110
Hopelessness, in case example,
  90–91
Humor, as behavioral intervention,
  98
Hypochondriasis, in case example,
  151

Identification with aggressor, as
  defense mechanism, 49–51,
  97–98, 115, 128, 142, 144–146
Impulse-control problems,
  psychodynamic approaches to,
  135–139
Inadequacy, as interfering factor in
  implementation of alternative
  behaviors, **103,** 105–106
Incompetence, presentation of as
  defensive maneuver, 29, 30, 32
Inhibition, in case examples, 116, 119
Interpersonal relationships. *See also*
    Couples therapy
  addressing of problem behaviors
    identified by others, 132–135
  dealing with response of others to
    behavioral change, 117–122
  reduction of contact or
    withdrawal from, 71
  time-limited dynamic
    psychotherapy and
    formulation of cyclical
    problematic, 9
  vicious cycle of interaction
    between intrapsychic states
    and, 8
Interpretation, as technique for
  addressing behavioral change,
  **42,** 43–51

Intrapsychic conflicts. *See also* Conflict
  behavioral scripts and, 96
  negative affects from behavioral change and, 112–113
  patient resistance to therapist's suggestions and, 32
  psychodynamic formulation of factors contributing to problematic behavior and, 60–61
  somatic preoccupations with trauma and, 151
  unassertiveness as focus of psychodynamic psychotherapy and, **14**, 15, 18, 19, 23
Intrapsychic states, and interpersonal relationships, 8
Irritability, as posttraumatic symptom, 149–151

Learning model, and phobic behavior as outcome of trauma, 148
Limit setting
  collaborative approach to alternative behaviors and, 88–91
  problems with setting limits with children, 127–135, 138
  response of others to behavioral change and, 118

Marriage, and couples' problems, 123–127
Meanings, of problematic behavior, 60, **74**, 76–79
Medications, recommending, prescribing, and monitoring of in psychoanalytic treatment, 7

Mentalization
  in case example, 134
  self-observational capacity and, 73–74
  as technique for addressing behavioral change, **42**, 52–53
  unassertiveness as factor contributing to behavior problems and, **14**, 16–17, 18, 20, 22, 23
  time-limited dynamic psychotherapy and, 9–10
Metaphors
  in case example, 137
  process of self-observation and, 74, 80–81
Monitoring
  of factors interfering in implementation of alternative behaviors, 102, **103**
  of medications, 7
  of scripts for alternative behaviors, 94
Motivation, in case example, 91–92

Narcissistic injury, in case example, 108
Negotiation, of differences between partners' needs and wishes, 124
Neutrality, and focus on behavioral change in psychoanalysis, **2**, 3

Panic attacks
  in case examples, 5, 29
  diary and self-monitoring of, 69
Panic disorder, in case example, 57
*Panic-Focused Psychodynamic Psychotherapy—eXtended Range* (Busch et al. 2012), ix–x

Parenting
   in case examples, 37–38, 80,
      84–85, 88–90, 138
   problematic behavior in response
      to trauma and, 146–147
   problems in setting limits with
      children and, 127–132, 138
Passive aggression, as defense
   mechanism, 15–16, 46–47
Patient(s), and adverse impacts of
   psychodynamic approaches on
   therapeutic relationship, 28–35
Personality difficulties, and
   unassertiveness as factor in
   behavior problems, **14**, 16
Phobic behavior, as outcome of
   trauma, 147–149
Posttraumatic stress disorder
   (PTSD), in case example, 149
Pragmatic psychodynamic
   psychotherapy (PPP), 4–5,
   8–9
Problematic behaviors. *See also*
   Alternative behaviors;
   Behavioral change; Phobic
   behavior; Self-destructive
   behavior
   addressing of issues identified by
      others, 132–135
   clarification and confrontation as
      core techniques for, 43
   context, fantasies, and emotions
      triggering anger and, 79–81,
      83
   developmental events and, 76
   examination of context, affects,
      and meanings of, 60, **74**
   examination of multiple
      contributors to, 84–85
   identification of behaviors as, 43,
      56–60
   impulse-control issues and,
      135–139
   methods for addressing common
      forms of, **125**
   psychodynamic formulation of
      factors contributing to, 60–61
   recurrence of, **113**, 116–117
   traumatic experiences and, 76,
      **143**
Procrastination, and identifying
   circumstances, feelings, and
   meanings of problematic
   behavior, 76–79, 81
Psychoanalysis, and psychoanalytic
   theory. *See also* Psychodynamic
   approaches
   behavioral change as aid to goals
      of, 10, **11**
   changing views on behavioral
      interventions in, 4–6
   identification of factors
      contributing to behavioral
      problems, viii–ix, 13
   potential adverse effects of
      targeting behavioral change
      in, vii, 1–4, 27, **28**, 68
   tools and techniques for
      addressing behavioral change
      in, 6–11, **42**
Psychodynamic approaches, to
   behavioral change. *See also*
   Alternative behaviors;
   Behavioral change; Problematic
   behaviors; Psychoanalysis;
   Psychodynamic formulation
   clarification and confrontation as
      techniques in, 42–43
   collaborative approach for
      identifying alternative
      behaviors, 88–92
   countertransference and, 53–54

Psychodynamic approaches, to
    behavioral change (*continued*)
  dealing with response of others to
    behavioral change in,
    117–122
  defense mechanisms and, 46–51
  dynamic factors contributing to
    problematic behavior, 81–83
  factors interfering with
    performance of alternative
    behaviors and, 101–110
  framework for targeting of behav-
    ioral change in, 55–71, 84–85
  free association and, 41–42
  identification of behavioral effects
    of developmental and
    traumatic events, 76
  identification of circumstances,
    feelings, and meanings of
    behavior, 76–79
  identification of context, fantasies,
    and emotions triggering
    anger, 79–81
  impulse-control problems and,
    135–139
  interpretation as technique in,
    43–46
  irritability as posttraumatic
    symptom and, 149–151
  marital or couples' problems and,
    123–127
  mentalization skills and, 52–53
  phobic behavior as outcome of
    trauma and, 147–149
  problematic parental behavior in
    response to trauma and,
    146–147
  problems identified by others and,
    132–135
  problems with setting limits with
    children and, 127–132
  repetition of traumatic
    experiences and, 143–144
  scripts for alternative behaviors
    and, 87, **88**, 92–99
  self-observational capacity and,
    73–76
  somatic preoccupations with
    trauma and, 151–153
  trauma and identification with
    aggressor, 144–146
  understanding of factors
    impeding behavioral change
    and, 13–24
  working with transference in,
    51–52
  working through as technique in,
    53
Psychodynamic formulation
  in case examples, 17–23, 30
  definition of, 14
  dynamic factors contributing to
    problematic behavior and
    development of, 81–83
  homework and development of
    written, 69–70
  of intrapsychic conflicts, defenses,
    and developmental factors in
    problematic behaviors, 60–61
Psychotherapy. *See* Behavior therapy;
    Cognitive-behavioral therapy;
    Couples therapy; Pragmatic
    psychodynamic psychotherapy;
    Psychodynamic approaches;
    Time-limited dynamic
    psychotherapy

Reaction formation, as defensive mech-
    anism, 15–16, 18, 47–49, 63
Rebellious reactions, as interfering
    factor in alternative behaviors,
    **103**, 106–108

Recurrence, of problematic behavior, **113,** 116–117
Reflective functioning (RF), unassertiveness and deficits in mentalization, 16
Rejection, fear of in case example, 115
Repetition, of traumatic experiences, 143–144
Repression, and traumatic sequelae, 142
Rescue, fantasies of, 108
Resistance
    countertransference and, 37
    forms of in implementation of alternative behaviors, 102
    therapeutic relationship and, 32–33
Response, of others to behavioral change, 117–122
Rigidity, and setting of limits with children, 128

Sadomasochistic interaction, in case example, 119
Scaffold, as metaphor for development of self-observational capacities, 74
Scripts
    alternative behaviors and, 87, **88,** 92–99, 109
    behavioral interventions and, 9
    homework and, 70
Self, and unassertiveness as factor in behavior problems, **14**
Self-destructive behavior
    repetition of traumatic experiences and, 143
    unassertiveness and, 15
Self-esteem
    impulse-control problems and, 135
    view of behavioral change as threat to, 106
Self-observational capacity, development of, 73–76
Separation anxiety, in case example, 29
Sexual behaviors, and impulse-control problems, 135
Somatic symptoms
    in case examples, 58, 103
    traumatic sequelae and, 142, 151–153
Substance abuse, and impulse-control problems, 135
Subtypes, of interpretations, 44
Suggestion, and avoidance of focus on behavioral change in psychoanalysis, vii, 1–2
Symptom substitution, and avoidance of focus on behavioral change in psychoanalysis, **2,** 3–4

Therapeutic alliance, and resistance of patient to therapist's suggestions, 32, 40
Therapeutic relationship, potential adverse impact of psychodynamic approaches to behavioral change on, **2,** 4, 28–35
Time-limited dynamic psychotherapy (TLDP), and approach to behavioral change, 9–10
Transference
    in case examples, 65, 106–107
    interpretation of as technique for addressing behavioral change, **42,** 44, 51–52
    potential adverse impacts of psychodynamic approaches on, **29,** 32, 33, 35, 40
    behavioral change as aid to psychoanalytic goals and, 10

Traumatic experiences
    assertiveness and, 14–15
    contribution of to problematic behaviors, 76, 142, **143**
    identification with aggressor as defense, 144–146
    irritability as symptom of, 149–151
    phobic behavior as outcome of, 147–149
    problematic parental behavior in response to, 146–147
    repetition of, 143–144
    somatic preoccupations in response to, 151–153
Triggers, of angry behavior, 79–81

Videotape, and process of self-observation, 74, 80

Wachtel, P. L., 3–4, 8, 9
Working through, as technique for addressing behavioral change, **42,** 53
Writing, of scripts, 94